THE FANTASY FOOTBALL BLACK BOOK
2021 Edition

By: Joe Pisapia
@JoePisapia17

Featuring
Mike Tagliere @MikeTagliereNFL
Kyle Yates @KyleYNFL
Michael F. Florio @MichaelFFlorio
Andrew Erickson @AndrewErickson
Nate Hamilton @DomiNateFF
Derek Brown @DBro_FFB
Scott Bogman @BogmanSports
Chris Meaney @chrismeaney
Kate Magdziuk @FFballblast
Lauren Carpenter @stepmomlauren
Chris McConnell @WizardOfRoto
Mike Randle @RandleRant
Billy Wasosky @BillyWaz88
Edited by Aaron Pags @FantasyTriage

D1377911

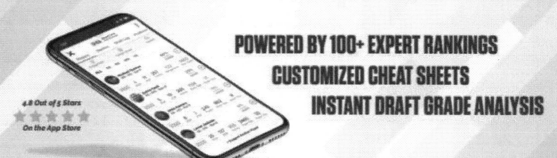

RPV CHEAT SHEETS
NOW AVAILABLE!

Want all the RPV for every format on one easy to reference cheat sheet PDF file? Plus, <u>FREE</u> updates sent in July & Aug!?

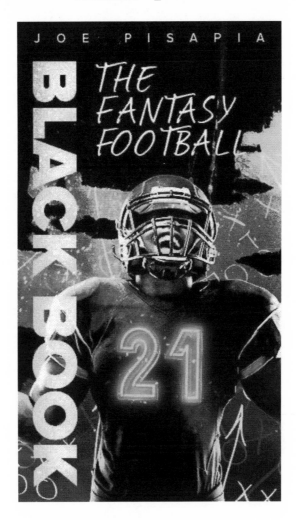

Send $5 to:
PayPal: <u>fantasyblackbook@gmail.com</u>
or
Venmo: @FantasyBlackBook
Be sure to write:
"Cheat Sheets" & add your <u>email address</u> in the comments!

About the Authors:

Joe Pisapia (@JoePisapia17 Twitter, @fantasyblackbook IG) *Joe is the author of the #1 best-selling Fantasy Black Book Series on Amazon and creator of the revolutionary player evaluation tool Relative Position Value (RPV). He's the host of the FantasyPros Fantasy Football Podcast, Leading Off Podcast, and Betting Pros Podcast. For television, Joe is currently the host of: "Diamond Bets (MLB)" & "Fantasy GameDay (NFL)" on SportsGridTV. Joe is a former radio host for Sirius/XM Fantasy Sports Radio and won the Fantasy Sports Radio Show of The Year Award (FSGA 2016). He frequently appears on CBS TV NY on The Sports Desk Show.*

Mike Tagliere *is the Lead Writer for FantasyPros.com, where you can find what some would call his weekly novel during the season, titled "The Primer." That is where Tagliere writes an entire paragraph on every player from every game, and best of all, it's free to read the whole 30-plus thousand-word piece. He also co-hosts the FantasyPros Football Podcast with Joe Pisapia and Kyle Yates. Ruler of Joey P's domain. Najee Harris truther. #AlwaysJulio. Dan Harris' best friend.*

Kyle Yates *is a Fantasy Analyst for FantasyPros. He's a co-host of the FantasyPros Football Podcast, the Host of The FantasyPros Dynasty Football Podcast, and is a Featured Writer. He can be found on Twitter @KyleYNFL.*

Michael F. Florio *can be found talking fantasy football on the NFL Network, NFL fantasy podcast, and on NFL.com. You can also hear him on SiriusXM Fantasy on RotoBaller Radio and RotoBaller.com. Before moving to LA to work for the NFL, he lived in NYC and held several different positions in the fantasy industry and has written for a wide variety of publications, including The Athletic, The Associated Press, and many others! When not drafting, talking, or writing fantasy football, he usually tries different food spots with his wife, Nicolette, or at the dog park with the cutest dog, Cali!*

Andrew Erickson *has been in fantasy football content space since 2017, but he finally "broke out" in 2020 when he caught the eyes of the nerds over at Pro Football Focus. Erickson signed a lucrative deal with the data provider and now rests his laurels on living life by his 6 Fs. Family, Friends, Food, Fitness, and Fantasy Football. There's a seventh F, but the editors took it out. Use your imagination :)*

Nate Hamilton *is the NFL Fantasy Analyst for The Game Day. This is his 4th-consecutive year writing for The Fantasy Football Black Book. Want to interact with Nate? Follow him on Twitter @DomiNateFF.*

Scott Bogman *has been in the Fantasy Sports industry since 2014, co-hosting Fantasy Football, Fantasy College Football, Fantasy Baseball, and Fantasy Basketball shows for In This League. Bogman also contributes to Sports Grid, CFB Winning Edge, and Linestar. This will be his 3rd year contributing rookie profiles and 2nd covering IDPs for the Black Book. You can find his work by following him on Twitter @BogmanSports or check out the In This League Patreon at Patreon.com/ITLArmy!*

Kate Magdziuk *is a co-founder of BallBlast Football, co-host of the BallBlast Fantasy Football Podcast, and this is her second season contributing to the Fantasy Football Black Book. In addition, she works full-time as an editorial coordinator with Vox Media for DraftKings Nation, formally transitioning from working as a full-time nurse to a full-time role in sports journalism last fall. She's previously worked as a contributor for NBC Sports Rotoworld, 4for4 Football, and RotoViz and is a member of the FSWA. Follow her on Twitter @FFballblast.*

Lauren Carpenter *graduated from the University of Missouri with a Bachelor of Journalism and is a fantasy football writer and analyst for the Fantasy Footballers, FantasyPros, NBCSports EDGE, and Football Guys. She combined her love of sports with her passion for writing to contribute to the fantasy football space. You can find her on social media @stepmomlauren, and you can find all of her work on her website stepmomlauren.com.*

Derek Brown can be found at the one-stop-shop for DFS, Fantasy, and betting content site Fade the Noise (FTN), with his work spread across FTNDaily.com, FTNFantasy.com, and FTNBets.com. His weekly podcast, Fade the Chalk, is available on all podcast streaming platforms, including Apple. Before going full-time at FTN, you could find his previous guest appearances on SiriusXM and DK Sweat. He was a finalist for the Fantasy Sports Writers Association DFS writer of the year award in 2020. Follow Derek on Twitter @DBro_FFB.

Chris Meaney is an award-winning sports writer, producer and host. He's Head of Content at Fade The Noise and the host of Mean Streets, FTN FAAB Cast, Fantasy Hockey Picks & Bets and FTN Live where he covers NFL, MLB, NHL & NBA from a fantasy sports and betting perspective. Meaney has been working in the in the fantasy sports industry for 10 years plus years making pit stops at The Athletic, The Fantasy Footballers, Anthem Sports & Entertainment, Fantrax, TQE, NBA Fantasy, LineStarApp, Newcap Radio and more.

Chris McConnell is a 16-year fantasy sports veteran and the host of the RotoBros Fantasy Football Podcast. Chris also runs the RotoBros Fantasy Advice Chat on Discord and hosts the weekly live show FSA Live in the FSA Fantasy Sports Advice & Analysis Facebook group. Self-proclaimed Chairman of the "RBDM" (Running Backs Don't Matter) community, Chris is a frequent guest on Sirius XM Fantasy Sports Radio and contributing partner at FleaFlicker.com. Residing in Georgia, Chris is a diehard Atlanta sports fan.

Billy Wasosky is an accomplished high-stakes fantasy football player who has been playing for 33 years. He was inducted into the NFFC Hall of Fame in 2014 and is well known for his successes in standard, auction, and draft champion formats. In 2019, he co-owned championships in both the NFFC Playoff Contest and the NFFC Diamond league, was 2nd overall in the 2013 Fantasy Football Players Championship, and was the overall champion in the 1995 Sporting News Fantasy Football Championship. His career high stakes winnings exceed $425,000.

Mike Randle (@RandleRant) covers NFL wagering for the Action Network, hosts the weekly RotoViz Fantasy Football Mailbag, and is the Editor-in-Chief of the PlayerProfiler Fantasy Football Draft Kit. In addition, he has covered Fantasy Football for LastWordOnNFL, RotoUnderworld, FantasyPros, Dynasty Trade Calculator, and FanSided.

Travis Sumpter has been playing fantasy football since 2011. Always a helping hand in the industry and am always willing to offer advice—Father of three beautiful boys, Evan, Adler, and Kaleb. When the pandemic hit, I took more to fantasy and got more involved in the FFC(Fantasy Football Community. Writer, Podcaster, Contributor, Co-Social Media Manager for Truth Serum Football. I started my journey with the help of Chris Pinto from Fantasy First Rounders Live (@FantasyFRLive) and Ben, Jay, and Steve (@TotalForesight). Thank Joey Fickle and Jordan Thomas from Truth Serum Football. I want to dedicate my portion of this to my beautiful wife Lindsay, my rock and biggest supporter. Follow myself (@tjsumpter55) and our group Truth Serum Football. (@TruthSerumFF)

Aaron Pags is a Featured Fantasy Football Writer for FantasyPros. He is a multi-sport Black Book contributor. He has written NFL Gambling advice for Razzball and currently hosts (w/ Nate Marcum) Bullpen Games, a fantasy baseball podcast. His sons, Tucker and Henry, aren't old enough to read this yet, but they will definitely add some color to the pages...literally! Follow Aaron for all things fantasy sports on Twitter @FantasyTriage.

TABLE OF CONTENTS

INTRODUCTION

This time last year, the world was in chaos and certainly there were more important things than football to be worried about. As I sit here, ready to release the 19th Fantasy Black Book, I'm overcome with a sense of relief. The relief that we're back to a place where we can worry about fantasy football again. We sometimes take for granted how lucky we are to have such seemingly trivial pastimes rule so much of our lives. My hope for everyone is that as we regain this sense of normalcy, without losing hold of the perspective we've been given over the last calendar year. I love the fantasy football community, and most of the time I REALLY like it as well. Sure, like every workplace there are challenges, but when the draft dust settles, there's no place I'd rather be than in the trenches, working with great people, covering the game I love.

11 years ago, I started this book journey with zero expectations. It spiraled into a radio journey, a TV journey and a broadcast career that I never planned on, but consider myself very lucky to have had so many opportunities to work with so many incredible people, from whom I have learned so much. The one constant all these years is the desire to do good work. I'm proud of The Black Book brand. I'm humbled by the talented individuals who are excited to be a part of it every year. Most importantly, I am grateful to the readers, listeners and supporters that have made this journey possible.

I say it every year, but it's true, this is the best edition of the Fantasy Football Black Book we have ever produced. The list of contributors speaks for itself, and our collective passion for the game leaps off the page. It's my goal to make every edition more comprehensive and useful than the last. The 2021 version will be tough to top (but we will, because that's what we do).

For those trying the Black Book for the first time, our goal is to be that one reference for all of your leagues. It's not a draft guide from the magazine rack. It's a system, a strategy and a season long companion for all of your leagues. Relative Position Value will change the way you draft, manage and play your leagues. If you're a returning member of #TeamBlackBook, welcome back!

Either way, thank YOU for making us the place you begin your 2021 fantasy football journey!

Joe

The 2021 Edition is dedicated to:
My two daughters, who picked every single NFL game
last year and ended in a tie with each other!
I'm so glad you are starting to love football Sundays!

SUNDAY, AUGUST 15, 2021
10:00am - 4:00pm
320 Market Avenue, Canton, Ohio 44702

Tickets Available online:
thefantasyfootballexpo.com

—— $10 / person ——

Chapter 1

RELATIVE POSITION VALUE (RPV)

Joe Pisapia

"The format and style of your league dictates the value of a player more than the talent of that player."

Another season, another onslaught of everyone's rankings, tiers and TOP 100 lists. Woohoo! #Sarcasm.

It's not enough...not even close. Rankings are a start, tiers are a step up (TOP 100, 300, whatever Lists are useless). Quantified rankings and tiers, now that's a strategy. In a landscape where opinions are bountiful, actual strategy is grossly under covered, underdiscussed, and underdelivered upon. That's not how the Black Book rolls. We give you all of it.

As I always say, well-educated and well-informed opinions are useful to an extent; otherwise, I wouldn't hire people to work with me on the Black Book. But that's just the beginning of a winning preparation process, while for most of the people you'll be playing against, it will be where their preparation ends.

NEVER mistake information and well-informed opinion for strategy. They're not, nor will it ever, be the same thing.

The sad part is that basically all that's out there is Fantasy Expert X's "Top 100," or Fantasy Expert Y's "Tiered Rankings" or Fantasy Expert Z's "Projections"? Don't get me started on those projection truthers, who never show accountability for their faulty computer software when things go awry. I don't know about you, but I don't want to live and die on hypotheticals alone. You need a cross section of these tools with an overriding, simple system, built in reality to truly understand how to approach each of your leagues.

Chances are you're playing in multiple leagues, with a myriad of different rules and scoring. That's why I created **Relative Position Value (RPV)**, the one tool to rule them all.

Rankings are what's out there, but QUANTIFIED Rankings are what RPV is all about. How much better is one player than another in a certain format? How drastic of a drop-off is there, not just player to player, but tier to tier? RPV can tell you.

RPV will automatically create player tiers -- and *define* them. It will also tell you how strong or weak a position player pool is, as a whole, entering a season. RPV is completely adaptable and adjustable to all league styles, depths and scoring systems. It's the single most useful player evaluation system available to fantasy owners and perhaps one of the easiest to grasp. I like simple and effective. RPV is both.

Year over year, this chapter won't change too much, because RPV is the foundation of the Black Book series. However, NFL players run fundamental drills in training camp, so if you're returning to RPV, consider this your return to fundamentals for the season and revisiting the basics that make you successful.

For those new to the Black Book series, RPV will have you seeing fantasy value in a whole new light. While other value-based drafting systems exist, they don't go far enough, nor do they separate the positions on a roster into subsets the way RPV does.

RB isn't a position, but RB1 is. (More to come on this later.) RPV is a more comprehensive and applicable system than any other thing you'll find out there.

STRIKING A BALANCE

Rankings are cute and wonderful debate fodder. However, it doesn't matter that Player A is ranked two slots above Player B on some "experts' board."

What REALLY matters is how much more productive Player A is than Player B -- and how much better they are than the other options at their position. Projections can be helpful, but not relied upon solely. When's the last time projectionists were held accountable (or held themselves accountable) for their many failures? The answer is hardly ever. Projections can have their place when you couple them with reality.

RPV compiles projections, previous season stats and three-year averages (when applicable) before weighing them to create a Black Book Point Total. That number is ALWAYS format-specific and is historically more reliable than projections alone, hence the success of the Black Book series. When it comes to rookies or young players, clearly we must rely more heavily on projections but use a cross-section to do so.

Now, what happens next to that Black Book Point Totals? Although I won't give away how I weigh them, I happily will give away the RPV formula: It's how we are going to proceed with a better understanding of fantasy football throughout the rest of the Black Book. RPV may challenge your perspective -- or quite possibly affirm feelings you've always had but now can see in black and white. Plus, once you have the formula, you can scale your own RPV for whatever insane scoring system you may be playing in, and you know who you are!

RPV IN THEORY

"RB isn't a position, BUT RB1 is!"

Considering a base of a 12-team league with two active RBs each week, a group of 24 running backs is a good starting point to grasp the RPV concept. However, it's NOT how we're going to truly utilize the tool.

Over 17 weeks in 2019, Christian McCaffrey led all PPR running backs with 471 pts for PPR scoring. Austin Ekeler ranked fourth with 309 pts. The 12th-best running back was Chris Carson at 236, and the 24th was David Montgomery with 170.

So, how much more valuable is each one of these guys compared to the other? Before we get ahead of ourselves, let's first see the formula in action.

The Fantasy Black Book formula is more complicated than the "basic" version I will present to you here. At the core, the way to determine the RPV -- or the percentage in which a player is better than the fantasy league average -- is:

(Individual Player Point Value – Fantasy League Average of the Position) ÷ Fantasy League Average of the Position = RPV

So, what is "Fantasy League Average?" Well, every league has a different number of teams and a varying number of active players at a given position. Some have 1RB/3WR/1FLEX, others play 2QB/2RB/3WR, and the list goes on and on.

The Fantasy League Average is a position's average production, based on the depth of your league. For example, if your league has 12 owners and starts 2RB every week, the RB pool is 24. If the top player scored 250 points and the 24th scored around 120, the fantasy league's scoring average is likely somewhere around 185 points. All players who score above this mark are "Positive RPV" players. The ones below are "Negative RPV."

Fantasy sports is a simple game of outscoring your opponents as frequently as possible from as many active positions as you can. The more your team lives in the "Positive," the greater your chances are week-to-week. It's like playing the odds in Texas hold'em. If you have a strong starting hand, the odds are in your favor. Sure, you may take some bad beats, but more often than not, the percentages will play in your favor.

Here's the trick! Even though there are 24 running backs, almost every team will likely have **one true RB1**, which means RB1 is its own unique scoring position. Rather than create a Fantasy League Average for 24 overall backs, it's more applicable to separate RB1s and RB2s into their own private groups and create an individual fantasy league average for each.

Now that we understand Fantasy League Average, let's get more specific. Last year, Alvin Kamara scored **336** (half PPR) pts. The Fantasy League Average (or FLA) at RB1 (top 12) in that scoring was **242** pts.

Subtract that FLA from Kamara's 336, then divide by that same FLA (242 pts) using the simple formula:

Relative Position Value of +38% RPV: [336-242] ÷ 242 = 38%.

Alvin Kamara was a +38% RPV better than the Fantasy League Average RB1 in 2020.

That means Kamara was 38% more productive than the average RB1 in fantasy leagues in that particular half PPR scoring. That's substantial! That means something!

If we took the RPV of running back as a whole over the top 24, Kamara's RPV would jump to a whopping +65% RPV, because the Fantasy League Average would be just 204 pts.

BUT we don't do that, because he'll be stacking up, head-to-head, against other RB1s most weeks in theoretical terms against other RB1 slots on other rosters. Calculating RB1s and RB2s as their individual positions gives a much more accurate depiction of a player's value, hence what makes RPV better than other value-based systems.

Are you in a 14-team league? Then use the top 14 to establish RB1 RPV. In a 10- team league? Adjust that way. The deeper the league, the more difficult it is to create an RPV advantage. The shallower the league, the less disparity you'll find (especially at WR). Therefore, you have more options to construct your roster in different ways. Have a wacky scoring system? Doesn't matter. RPV formula covers everything.

Below is the **Final RPV** for RB1s and RB2s from the end of 2020. You'll see not only the positive but also the negative side of RPV. The avoidance of over drafting/overspending on players that can't really supply you with "positive" production or as I like to say, 'move the needle". This clears the path to success. You will also see as we go on how to create an RPV advantage.

2020 FINAL RB RPV for RB1 and RB2 (Half PPR scoring)

RB 1 HALF PPR				RB 2 HALF PPR		
Player	FPTS	RPV		Player	FPTS	RPV
1 Alvin Kamara (NO)	336.3	39%		1 Melvin Gordon III (DEN)	182.4	10%
2 Derrick Henry (TEN)	323.6	34%		2 Kenyan Drake (LV)	179.7	8%
3 Dalvin Cook (MIN)	315.8	30%		3 Mike Davis (ATL)	177	6%
4 David Montgomery (CHI)	237.8	-2%		4 Ronald Jones II (TB)	172.3	4%
5 Aaron Jones (GB)	235.4	-3%		5 Chris Carson (SEA)	169.3	2%
6 Jonathan Taylor (IND)	234.8	-3%		6 D'Andre Swift (DET)	166.8	0%
7 James Robinson (JAC)	225.9	-7%		7 David Johnson (HOU)	163	-2%
8 Josh Jacobs (LV)	214.8	-11%		8 Nyheim Hines (IND)	161.7	-3%
9 Nick Chubb (CLE)	199.7	-18%		9 J.K. Dobbins (BAL)	159.5	-4%
10 Kareem Hunt (CLE)	199.5	-18%		10 Clyde Edwards-Helaire (KC)	158	-5%
11 Ezekiel Elliott (DAL)	197.7	-18%		11 Miles Sanders (PHI)	156.4	-6%
12 Antonio Gibson (WAS)	184.2	-24%		12 JD McKissic (WAS)	151	-9%

The first obvious takeaway from last year was there was a tremendous drop off after the top 3 RBs, from +30% RPV to -2%RPV. There were the teams with the elite RBs and then there was everyone else. With time missed from Christian McCaffrey and Saquon Barkley, plus disappointing play from Ezekiel Elliott, RB1 took a significant hit. If they all rebound in '21 and Nick Chubb plays a full season, these percentages will surely get tighter. RB2 was much more forgiving, as usual. There was less separation in terms of their overall productivity. RPV is not only a great tool to use in drafts but also analyzing what's happening around the league.

How is RPV crafted for 2021?

I use a weighted system of projections, previous season stats and 3-year averages/college stats when applicable for veterans and rookies. That creates the fantasy point totals for a player, then I use the RPV formula to compare them to each other in their respective tier. For clarity, RB1's with low/negative RPV should be taken before RB2's with high RPV because the RPV is comparative to their tier.

So, how can the fantasy player exploit RPV?

By having a high-end RB1 and then drafting ANOTHER RB1 as your RB2, you have "frontloaded" the position and created an area of strength.

The BIGGEST mistake fantasy owners make in any sports in "filling their roster for positions," instead of filling their roster with talent and strength.

When you fill your roster for positions, you get a mediocre .500 team. When you fill your roster with strength, you have an advantage over the rest of the field. As long as you can responsibly fill the other positions and avoid Negative RPV as often as possible, that roster strength can carry your season.

With more NFL teams adapting backfield committees, the true starting running backs are worth more than ever in standard formats. That especially goes for the RB1s who get goal-line carries and the bulk of touches. In PPR, you can build the same strength of front-loading WR1s as you can with RB1s, then make up ground later by buying running backs in bulk with upside. The tough sell there is the difference between definitive running back touches as opposed to expected wide receiver catches. One is frankly more reliable on a weekly basis.

The same could be said for Superflex/2QB leagues. By "frontloading" elite QB play, you simultaneously create a team RPV strength and weaken the pool for the other owners. RPV shows you how stark the value can be position-to-position. Some will bottom out at -10% while others will be -20%. With middle-tier receivers, you'll see little advantage to be gained.

RPV is the ultimate tool to truly define talent and, even more importantly, where the drop-off in talent lies. Rankings are biased. RPV is honest.

Obviously, every league will be different. Flex players and OP (offensive player) slots will change values a bit, but the RPV theory holds in **EVERY LEAGUE and EVERY FORMAT**! It just needs to be adjusted according to each league's specifications. In the Black Book, I've done much of the work for you, but you must be sure to adjust the RPV for your league(s) quirky scoring wrinkles if you are going to truly achieve ultimate success.

Now that we've outlined RPV, let's dive deeper.

RPV IN PRACTICE (Draft and Trades)

Last year, so many folks asked, "How does the Black Book determine its RPV?"

The Black Book takes a combination of 3-year averages (when applicable/available), previous season stats, and the upcoming season projections, creating a hybrid point total for each player that then gets utilized within the RPV equation.

For rookies, clearly there is no track record from which to work to create that number. Therefore, I use a composite of projected stats from a few choice entities, their college statistical profile, and their potential use in their new team system in order to create each rookie's point total for the RPV formula.

With so many new styles of fantasy football, it's crucial to understand the value of each position in your league.

For example, I prefer PPR (point per reception) setups that play a lineup consisting of QB, RB, RB/WR, WR1, WR2, WR3, TE, K, 5 IDP and an OP slot (which can be a QB) or a second mandatory QB spot.

If a quarterback is the most important skills entity in *real* football, I want my fantasy experience to mirror that truth. The RPV for this kind of league is different than a standard league. Teams play 2 QBs every week, therefore QBs become the equivalent of the RB1/RB2 RPV I just laid out in the last section.

Another big adjustment: Since I technically only have to start 1 RB, the talent pool is adjusted back into a "one large group of running backs" theory. Possession WRs and big playmakers garner attention. This is a perfect example of why a tool like RPV is so necessary. If I were to use the standard old rankings from a website or a magazine in this format, I would get crushed.

Now more than ever, there is no "one ranking system" that will be useful to you in any format. Ignore these Top 100 lists and nonsense like that -- and instead focus on the true value and weight of the player in *your* league. That's why RPV works.

The last best thing about RPV is the fact it strips away a lot of the hype and noise surrounding the athletes, as well as the fictional computer projections that can be misleading and downright destructive.

RPV is about understanding a player's value -- his ACTUAL value. Not what his value may be projected to be while you sit in last place wondering where you went wrong. The best way to evaluate a player is through a mixture of career averages, previous statistics and projections that are then weighed against the other players of the same position. NOT PROJECTIONS ALONE!

Using only last year's numbers will give you a great team … for last season. Using just projections will give you a great team … in theory. RPV will give you a great team in REALITY!

You can choose to be great at one spot or two, but if you are below-average at other places, your overall RPV will even out. You may find yourself managing a middle-of-the-road team. Being above-average in as many places as you can, even without a top-flight star, you will find yourself consistently out-producing your opponents. If you use RPV correctly, you may even find yourself above average in most places and great in others, which makes you the one to beat. It's the ability to adapt, adjust and understand that separates us. RPV is the difference-maker.

RPV can tell you not only how much better a player is than the average for his position, but also how much better he is than the next guy available at his position on the draft board. Understanding these RPV relationships is key in maximizing your positional advantage.

To illustrate this point and its application, let's take a draft-day example. It's your turn to pick, and you have openings to fill at WR and TE. The top available players on the board at each position look like this:

WR

- Player A: +15% RPV
- Player B: +10% RPV
- Player C: +8% RPV
- Player D: +7% RPV
- Player E: +5% RPV

TE

- Player F: +8% RPV
- Player G: -2% RPV
- Player H: -2% RPV
- Player I: -4% RPV
- Player J: -6% RPV

At first glance, you might be inclined to take Player A, who is a +15% better than the average at his position. All other things being equal, however, Player F is probably the better choice.

Even though he is only +8% better than the average, the drop-off between him and the next-best player at his position is 10 percentage points. That's a significant dip. If you take Player A now, Player F almost definitely won't be on the board when your next pick rolls around, and at best you'll be stuck with an average or below-average tight end.

If you take Player F now, however, you'll be on the right side of that 10% RPV advantage over the teams who haven't drafted a TE yet. You'll also probably lose out on Player A at WR, but you will still most likely get someone from the above list (Player C, D or E) -- all of whom are trading in the same RPV range and, more importantly, still in the positive. It may not sound like a big deal with mere percentage points, but it adds up the more you rise above or fall below the average RPV threshold.

By picking this way, you end up with a strong advantage at one position while remaining above average at the other. The alternative is to be above-average at one position and decidedly average or worse at the other. That's the reason so many fantasy owners fail. Usually, they base these decisions on the *name* of the player instead of his Relative Position Value. The same can be said when evaluating trades. You must look at what advantage you're gaining and potentially losing in each deal.

The owner who does that effectively has a distinct advantage. Remember, don't marginalize your strength!

Everyone has access to opinions, but now you have access to RPV.

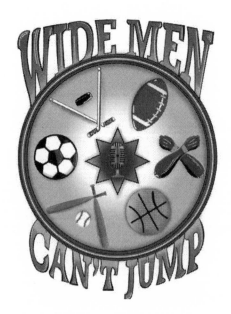

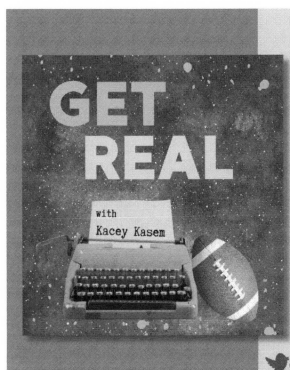

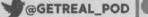 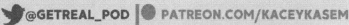

Chapter 2
Draft Strategy 2021

PPR DRAFT STRATEGY
Joe Pisapia

CORE ROSTER BUILDING 4 ROUND MOCK

	ROUND 1	ROUND 2	ROUND 3	ROUND 4
1	Christian McCaffrey	Allen Robinson	Antonio Gibson	Adam Thielen
2	Dalvin Cook	Keenan Allen	Darren Waller	Travis Etienne
3	Derrick Henry	George Kittle	Terry McLaurin	Lamar Jackson
4	Jonathan Taylor	Justin Jefferson	Chris Godwin	Clyde Edwards-Helaire
5	Alvin Kamara	Julio Jones	Najee Harris	Diontae Johnson
6	Saquon Barkley	Calvin Ridley	Amari Cooper	Dak Prescott
7	Nick Chubb	D.K. Metcalf	Miles Sanders	Kyler Murray
8	Ezekiel Elliott	A.J. Brown	Patrick Mahomes	Robert Woods
9	Davante Adams	Joe Mixon	Josh Allen	Michael Thomas
10	Travis Kelce	Austin Ekeler	David Montgomery	Mike Evans
11	Stefon Diggs	DeAndre Hopkins	D'Andre Swift	Chris Carson
12	Tyreek Hill	Aaron Jones	J.K. Dobbins	CeeDee Lamb

2021 PLAYER POOL OVERVIEW

Ah, the most popular format, the PPR. Although I recommend the .5 point version, the full PPR is the arcade version of fantasy football that we've grown to love over the last decade. The evolution of the NFL into a "pass first league" is now complete. That means there are more options at wide receiver than ever, and more running backs catching the ball out of the backfield. The TE position is going to make advances over the next year or so, with some tremendous emerging talents. It's still a player pool dominated by the all-purpose running backs at the top. However, doubling up on elite wide receivers is viable, as is waiting for underappreciated wide receiver talent. The key to this format is identifying players who could make the jump from WR2 to WR1, WR3 to WR 2 and so on and so forth. In 2019, the Black Book gave you Chris Godwin and DJ Moore. Last year, we gave you Calvin Ridley and D.K. Metcalf. In 2021, CeeDee Lamb, Terry McLaurin, Tee Higgins and Ja'Marr Chase are those likely names to make those jumps. When you hit on those talents and they jump a tier, it allows you to invest early in elite RB, QB and TE and still have solid WR talent on your roster.

12 TEAM LEAGUE DRAFT SLOT APPROACH

As I said, the top still belongs to the all-purpose RB studs. The middle of the first round is up for debate, but the clear value at the bottom of the draft is going to be elite WRs with high Relative Position Values. Doubling up with two creates an advantage, as does an elite WR with Travis Kelce. Team 11 in that mock, is where I want to live. Two great WRs, two solid RBs with upside and a roster that's now free to take a big QB or best player available after that. If you're going to take a big QB in the first four rounds, I would suggest applying the "WR Jumper Strategy" (the guys who can jump a tier I just discussed) and take your RB's early, with that Patrick Mahomes or Josh Allen selection.

SHALLOW (10 TEAM LEAGUE) VS. DEEP (14+TEAM) LEAGUE APPROACH

In 10 team leagues, I would definitely hit RB early and often. There's just such a favorable supply and demand ratio for wide receivers that you can afford to wait. In fact, you can justify the super elite QB picks as well in the first few rounds of a 10-team league for the same reason. There will be less RPV advantages in a pool of 10 starting QB's than 12.

When dealing with deeper PPR leagues, I'm very high and taking the value on the board, regardless of position. Build a core roster strength somewhere, then attack your roster deficiencies later on in the draft. The biggest mistake fantasy players make is trying to "fill their roster" instead of build greatness. You just have to have a good working knowledge of the player pool, and maybe find some ADP loopholes on your host site (players you think have upside, that are undervalued in ADP). In deeper formats, I would also prefer to focus on RB and WR, and be open to playing QB matchups by drafting more than one and a value later in the draft.

IF YOU COULD PICK YOUR DRAFT SLOT

I would always prefer to have an elite all-purpose RB to start which means a top pick, but in PPR give me the bottom of the draft. Let me prey on the players that get passed over and fall too far. Let me load up on multiple great players and spread my risk, while maintaining above average roster productivity.

PLAYERS OUTSIDE OF THE 4 ROUND MOCK

In some publications, you won't see Kyler Murray or Dak Prescott go in the first four rounds, and I think that's a mistake. They're dominant fantasy forces and protected by the rules of the NFL. If they should last in your draft to the 5th round, pounce. In rounds 5 and 6 I think it's a mistake to chase TEs that don't move the needle. T.J. Hockenson and Mark Andrews are nice, but league average TE. You are better off grabbing more WR depth and upside RBs, then take some shots on TE later. I'm very Ricky Bobby when it comes to TE, you're either first (Travis Kelce) or you're last (let them come to you).

HOW TO RUIN YOUR DRAFT

The quickest way to ruin your draft is to draft for need too soon. What you NEED is high end productivity from somewhere. There will be plenty of opportunity to draft for need later, but drafting greatness is basically relegated to the first few rounds of the draft. Shaping a great roster core is easy, dragging a mediocre roster core to greatness is very difficult.

SUPERFLEX DRAFT STRATEGY

Joe Pisapia

CORE ROSTER BUILDING 4 ROUND MOCK

	ROUND 1	ROUND 2	ROUND 3	ROUND 4
1	Christian McCaffrey	Lamar Jackson	Russell Wilson	Robert Woods
2	Dalvin Cook	Julio Jones	George Kittle	Mike Evans
3	Derrick Henry	Dak Prescott	Allen Robinson	CeeDee Lamb
4	Patrick Mahomes	Justin Jefferson	Austin Ekeler	Darrell Henderson
5	Jonathan Taylor	Calvin Ridley	Aaron Rodgers	Amari Cooper
6	Alvin Kamara	D.K. Metcalf	Keenan Allen	Matt Ryan
7	Josh Allen	A.J. Brown	Joe Mixon	J.K. Dobbins
8	Saquon Barkley	Aaron Jones	Chris Godwin	Tom Brady
9	Nick Chubb	DeAndre Hopkins	Terry McLaurin	David Montgomery
10	Ezekiel Elliott	Tyreek Hill	Darren Waller	Miles Sanders
11	Davante Adams	Stefon Diggs	Antonio Gibson	Justin Herbert
12	Travis Kelce	Kyler Murray	Najee Harris	Michael Thomas

2021 PLAYER POOL OVERVIEW

In 2021 superflex drafts, it's wise to hit QB and RB early and often. As tempting as many of the high end WRs may be, there is so much depth (especially in PPR scoring) to make up ground there later. Early QB selections also typically push the 1AWR/high end WR2s back a round or two, creating outstanding value. If you fall behind at QB and RB, you could be fighting an uphill battle. There are very few bell-cow running backs, but there are a few RBs worth taking risks in, such as Najee Harris and Joe Mixon.

12 TEAM LEAGUE DRAFT SLOT APPROACH

The top RB's should still go where they typically do within the top 5 picks, but if your QB scoring is extraordinarily favorable, then you can certainly push Patrick Mahomes, Josh Allen and Kyler Murray into that range. With a top 5 pick, you can easily go "Best Player Available" in rounds 2 or 3, or you can double down on a position and create an RPV advantage. For example, taking Christian McCaffrey at 1 overall then doubling up at QB with Lamar Jackson and Russell Wilson gives you an RPV advantage at RB and at QB1 and superflex/OP slot with a QB1 in Wilson there over a QB2. From the middle slots, you're more at the mercy of the board. The best approach is to take advantage of what falls to you that shouldn't. If you can snag Alvin Kamara, Saquon Barkley or Josh Allen, you are off to a good start. The second round will offer you the top tier WR most likely based on ADP, but be sure that you address QB by the time you leave the 6th round with two, if you should start RB/WR in rounds 1-2. From the bottom of the snake draft, you can make a few different approaches work. I love getting Travis Kelce and a QB (if you can pull that off), then let the pool come to you in rounds 3-4. To a certain extent, you can create a run by doubling up with a back-to-back QB, or RB or WR at the bottom, creating a supply demand issue. If you're going to double dip, do it at QB or WR. It's just a safe investment at that point, unless Nick Chubb slips farther than he should.

SHALLOW (10 TEAM LEAGUE) VS. DEEP (14+TEAM) LEAGUE APPROACH

Ironically, the shallower the league, the more aggressive I would be on top QBs. There is frankly more replacement value on the wire, and the depth of the wide receiver position is at an all-time high. You can make up ground there later on while getting your QB and RB situation strong early. In a deep league Superflex, it's imperative to let the value come to you. Ideally, you would like to come away with a top 7 QB and a high-end QB2. I would also make it a point to reach for a 3rd QB as insurance for injury and bye weeks. A decent 3rd QB in a deeper league can be extremely valuable to your roster.

IF YOU COULD PICK YOUR DRAFT SLOT

Personally, I would like to be at the top and get that elite RB, then settle my QBs, and go WR crazy later. The 7-spot in the mock is very strong too, taking a big QB, then a big WR and two upside RB's in rounds 3-4. I actually won the SuperFlex Flex League Championship in '19 with that strategy.

PLAYERS OUTSIDE OF THE 4 ROUND MOCK

After the first four rounds, there should be some strong quarterbacks still available such as: Kirk Cousins, Joe Burrow, Ryan Tannehill etc. The same cannot be said for running back, which falls off substantially. Wide receiver on the other hand is abundant. There are plenty of former #1's like JuJu Smith-Schuster, Odell Beckham and Kenny Gollday. There are also some great young talents like Ja'Marr Chase, Tee Higgins and Brandon Aiyuk. The point is, when you understand the player pool, the RPV advantages to be had and the way QB ADP suppresses WR ADP in a superflex, the draft is yours to control.

HOW TO RUIN YOUR DRAFT

Thinking there are enough quarterbacks around that you can make up ground later in the draft is a recipe for disaster. While there is some upside in the QB2 pool, there is also a ton of risk as well, not to mention a few QB's on the hot seat with youngsters nipping at their heels for playing time. The possibility of falling grossly behind the teams with solid QB play (which is typically steadier than that of the other positions in terms of weekly floor productivity) is a potential season killer. Don't let that happen to you.

STANDARD DRAFT STRATEGY

Nate Hamilton

CORE ROSTER BUILDING 4 ROUND MOCK

	ROUND 1	ROUND 2	ROUND 3	ROUND 4
1	Christian McCaffrey	Patrick Mahomes	George Kittle	Adam Thielen
2	Dalvin Cook	Allen Robinson	Josh Allen	Diontae Johnson
3	Derrick Henry	Julio Jones	J.K. Dobbins	CeeDee Lamb
4	Jonathan Taylor	Calvin Ridley	Anontio Gibson	Robert Woods
5	Nick Chubb	Justin Jefferson	Miles Sanders	Lamar Jackson
6	Saquon Barkley	D.K. Metcalf	Keenan Allen	Dak Prescott
7	Ezekiel Elliott	A.J. Brown	Darren Waller	Kyler Murray
8	Alvin Kamara	Najee Harris	Chris Godwin	Amari Cooper
9	Aaron Jones	Tyreek Hill	Chris Carson	Michael Thomas
10	Davante Adams	David Montgomery	Austin Ekeler	Terry McLaurin
11	Stefon Diggs	Joe Mixon	Clyde Edwards-Helaire	Mike Evans
12	Travis Kelce	DeAndre Hopkins	D'Andre Swift	Darrell Henderson

Standard Scoring

When something is titled "standard", it means that it's the typical example or it's regularly used. Each year that passes, "standard scoring" is anything but the standard in fantasy football. Today, the majority of fantasy players prefer to have a value attached to receptions. When you earn points for receptions, your league scoring format is considered to be a points-per-reception (PPR) scoring format.

If the majority of fantasy players are in some form of PPR leagues then that should be considered the standard and the current standard should be named something else. The word standard should be removed from our vocabulary in fantasy football. There should be types of PPR and non-PPR, but I digress.

2021 Player Pool Overview

In standard leagues, it's important to draft players that receive a healthy workload. Running backs that get a ton of carries is a great place to start. It's difficult to rely on pass-catching backs as you do not gain fantasy points with receptions. Luckily, in today's NFL, the majority of workhorse running backs are also great receiving options. This will help make your decisions easier if you find yourself in both PPR and standard leagues.

Everyone has their draft strategies, but I'd advise you to draft a top-tier running back in the first round if you can. Few running backs provide a safe floor with volume and efficiency, so you'll want to secure one of them on your roster before the pool dries up.

Regardless of position, you'll want to look for players who receive a heavy workload. For pass-catchers, look not only at target numbers but how they convert those opportunities into yards/touchdowns since the receptions alone will not provide you with fantasy points. If you are unable to draft one of the top-5 quarterbacks, you may want to aim for one that has rushing upside. This will give you a safe floor at the position since rushing yards will generate fantasy points.

DRAFT SLOT APPROACH

Picks 1-4: These picks should not be overthought. You have an opportunity to add one of the best running backs in the league to your fantasy team. Do it. You'll be watching a lot of the top-tier players fly off the boards as you wait what will feel like an eternity before your second pick. Having that safe, workhorse running back will make you feel better during this difficult time.

Your next two picks will be closer together so evaluate the draft board and go with the best receiver available unless there is still another running back who will see plenty of quality volume. If that's the case, I wouldn't blame you for starting your draft with two running backs. You can always draft a wide receiver with your third pick since your second and third picks will be close together.

With your fourth pick, assess your team and try to balance it out from a positional standpoint. You may want to make a move and get one of the remaining top-3 tight ends or quarterbacks if possible. If your team is already looking balanced, opt for the best player available.

Picks 5-8 The 2021 player pool should allow you to follow the advice for players with picks 1-4, at least for the first pick. As you can see in the mock draft that Joe and I did, the first nine picks were all running backs. Get yourself one of these elite running back options because they will not be there when it comes time for your second pick.

Since your picks will be more evenly separated, it may be best for you to take the best player available with your next few picks. Hopefully, it works out and creates a balanced foundation for the rest of the draft.

Focus on running backs and wide receivers with these core-building picks, but do not ignore if a top-tier tight end or quarterback is available in the middle of the fourth round.

Picks 9-12 At first glance, you may feel frustrated with landing a late first-round pick. You will likely miss out on the top-tier running backs, but there is a positive here. Your first two picks will be back-to-back or very close to it. This means that you can guarantee two top-12 players at their particular position to begin your draft. This is why drafting at or close to the turn is my favorite draft slot.

More often than not, your team will feel much better through the first two rounds than your league mate's teams with earlier picks. If you have a pick toward the end of the first round, hopefully, you are feeling much better about your draft slot now.

Depending on how you began your draft, you'll want to use your next two picks as a balancing act. If you haven't caught on already, balance with your early picks will allow you to draft the best player available the deeper you get into the draft. If you balance early, you won't have to spend any of your draft trying to play catch up on a specific position.

SHALLOW (10 TEAM LEAGUE) VS. DEEP (14+TEAM) LEAGUE APPROACH

When there are fewer people in your league, you will feel the temptation to either draft all the top running backs or wide receivers because they will be available to you. Fight that temptation. I mentioned this in last year's Fantasy Football Black Book. Although you could secure a fair share of top talented players in one position, you can't play them all at the same time. You'll be investing your valuable picks on someone that will spend time on your bench. When drafting the core of your team, focus on getting the top players from positions you know will be in your starting lineup every week. Balancing early will reduce the pressure in your draft pick decisions for the remainder of the draft.

In a deeper league, core building becomes even more important. When you have more people in your league, more players are drafted between your draft picks. Science!
You must look ahead and adjust according to how the majority are drafting. Having more league mates dramatically impacts the value of all players in the draft. If you see a run from a particular position of need leading up to your next pick, you'll want to get what you can in that position with that pick. If you do not react appropriately, you will miss out and you will not be satisfied with what will be available come time for your next pick.

By the end of your draft, even when executed perfectly, you may not feel thrilled about your team as a whole when you look back at it. Do not panic. The main reason for this is a result of the size of your league. Just look at the other teams and you'll quickly feel much better about your draft.

IF YOU COULD PICK YOUR DRAFT SLOT

All draft slots have their positives and negatives. The early draft picks will get one of the few best running backs in the league, but will have to wait a long time between picks. The middle picks are evenly spaced and create balance from a value standpoint. The picks closer to the turn will allow you to begin your draft with two high-end players, but like the early picks, you'll have many players taken off the board before your next pair of picks.

I tend to love the draft slots that are toward the end of the first round. I believe it's best to begin your draft and core building with two upper-echelon players. You have two picks close enough to one another that each time it's your turn to draft, you'll be drafting players in the same tier or very close to it.

PLAYERS OUTSIDE OF THE 4 ROUND MOCK

Every year players will drop in average draft position due to injury, aging, situational changes, etc... These are things you should pay close attention to. If you see that a certain player is being drafted later than they were last season, investigate why that is and use that information to decide on how much you currently value that player.

Josh Jacobs may still be drafted in the first four rounds in some drafts, but Joe and I felt his value is significantly impacted by the addition of Kenyan Drake to the Raiders' backfield.

James Robinson will not have the backfield to himself this year. The Jaguars drafted Clemson running back Travis Etienne with the 25th overall pick. The coaching staff is trying to peg Etienne as their 3rd-down back, but it's highly unlikely the first-round pick will not have a larger role carved out.

HOW TO RUIN YOUR DRAFT

Championships are not won at the draft, but they can be lost. The easiest way to ruin your draft is to invest heavily in a single position early on. I can't emphasize enough how important it is to have some semblance of balance in your roster with your early picks.

If you draft too many of one thing, you will be chasing the other positions the rest of the draft and beyond. You could find yourself in a predicament where you become so desperate for production out of the position you waited on. You may feel obligated to trade one of your higher drafted players for one of lesser value just to add balance to your roster. Be smart and balance your early core building picks so you do not find yourself in this position.

AUCTION /HIGH STAKES (NFFC) STRATEGY

Billy Wasosky

I would be willing to bet that almost everyone who has read this article has drafted in your standard "snake draft." The thought of getting your draft slot is something many of us look forward to, and if you are like me, you dream of ways to build a juggernaut around the Christian McCaffrey's and Dalvin Cooks of the world. Then you receive your draft slot, and you get to pick at 9. Ugh......your dreams now come crashing down, and you are hoping that the consensus 7th or 8th round overall pick fall in your lap, while your buddy who knows far less than you (in your mind anyhow), fell into the number one pick, and is doing his or her "CMac dance" and talking trash. The beauty of an auction is that you aren't bound to a specific spot, you don't have to worry about getting "sniped" one pick in front of you, and you can get all your "sleepers" in one draft. So, while snake drafts are fine (isn't drafting always great?), playing in an auction league takes everything to another level!

This article intends to share strategies that I feel apply to winning not only your local auction league but also playing in high-stakes auction leagues. All the auction leagues I currently play in are at the NFFC (National Fantasy Football Championship) at nfc.shgn.com/football. The NFFC offers online and live auctions ranging from $150 - $5,000 entries and has some of the best auction players in the entire country. While an online auction carries an unparalleled excitement to a snake draft, NOTHING compares to a live auction in New York or Las Vegas! Watching your friends bid up a player that you have no interest in, bidding $1 extra to try and squeeze a little more out of an owner (more on that later), winning the player you wanted for less than you had them projected for, etc. In a live auction, watching the expressions of everyone at the table, the trash-talking after a "bad" pick, ...it is simply the absolute best 2.5 - 3 hours you can spend assembling a team.

I'm assuming that if you bought this book, you have at least heard of auction drafting. However, if you haven't, here is a quick overview;

- The draft starts with team one nominating and goes down the line through team 12 (or however many teams you have, and then begins again at team one and repeats through 20 rounds). Your draft/nominating spot is of little to no importance in an auction.
- Each owner nominates any player/DST they want. Once a player/DST is nominated, anyone can bid higher (no less than $1 increments), just like an auction for antiques, cars, etc., the person who has the highest bid after the auctioneer says, "SOLD!" wins that player.
- Every team is provided $200 fictitious dollars to purchase 20 players.
- You must purchase 20 players, but you don't necessarily have to spend the whole 200 dollars (however, you can't "take it with you").

"EVERY PLAYER IS WORTH WHAT SOMEONE WILL PAY"
"THE LAST PLAYER IN A TIER, AND BEING FLEXIBLE"

A little over a month before writing this chapter, an autographed Tom Brady rookie card sold in an auction for roughly 2.25 million dollars! In its purest form, a football card is a photo, on a piece of cardboard, with someone's signature. While that price tag seems excessive to me, someone valued that card that much and is now proud. A fantasy football auction is similar...all it takes is for 2 (or more) people who want a player, and the bidding on that player can become fast and furious. However, in my experiences with auctions, what causes players to go much higher than their perceived value is SCARCITY. Here is an example:

You need an RB1, and all but one of the first ten consensus RBs are gone. Alvin Kamara sits on most people's boards is a top 3-5 RB in any format this upcoming season. You have plenty of money left, as does almost every other owner in your league. You have Alvin Kamara listed as a $52 RB. The bidding begins, and many in the room are bidding on him. The price climbs quickly to $50, and before you can blink, someone yells, "$55!" Then a "$56! $57!". You look at your sheet, and you have seconds to decide to raise the bid to $58 or lose out on a top 5 RB.

Auction players I admire very much are very strict with their auction values and will not go any higher than what they have on their respective sheets. What works best for me is being flexible, and if the market dictates, you need to spend more for certain players/positions. For example, if most WRs are going $3-$5 more than you anticipated, there will be value at other positions that you can take advantage of later in the auction at RB, QB, TE, etc.

STRATEGIES TO USE IN YOUR AUCTION

As you can already see, there are so many more variables that come into play in an auction draft than in a standard snake draft. I have probably done 40-50 auction drafts in my lifetime, and in every single one of them, I have taken something new away from each one. You are in on EVERY player (you can't make your pick at number 1, and then go to the bathroom and scan the board 23 picks later in an auction), so you have to be ready for anything. Since that is the case, incorporating quality strategies is often going to be paramount to your success. Here are some of the best strategies that I feel have worked for me;

MOCK OUT DIFFERENT SCENARIOS
I will often be on the plane flying to my drafts, in a hotel the morning of my auction, at a red light writing on a napkin, etc., mocking out my newest version of "my perfect auction." Of course, it changes daily as the news changes, and it is more challenging than winning Powerball to get the exact players you mapped out, but it is a perfect exercise, IMO. As I mentioned earlier, being FLEXIBLE (with both players and $ amounts) is the key.

NOMINATING PLAYERS
Some people believe in nominating players who you don't want (to make others spend their money). Some players believe in nominating players they want, so they can "get their guy." I think you have to do a combination of both and keep your competition guessing. If you play against good competition and don't mix it up, they will quickly figure you out and use it against you.

PRICE ENFORCING
This is by far the most fun strategy to implement in an auction. It is simply bidding $1 higher to make the other person spend $1 extra or bidding $1 higher because you feel the nominated player is grossly undervalued. But, can it backfire on you, and you get stuck with a player you had no intention of taking? Of course, it can! So I don't recommend you do it unless you are ready to own that player or are highly confident someone will be willing to pay $1 more.

"AVOID GOING ON TILT"
This is probably the most critical strategy. There will most likely be a point in the auction where you A) Get outbid for a player you wanted or B) You ended up spending a little too much on a player, and it put your remaining budget in a bind. The key is you need to shake it off, and QUICK! The alternative is that you dwell on that latest mishap, and it will most likely negatively affect what you do for the remainder of the draft. Whether you are ready or not, someone will nominate a player in another few seconds. So it would help if you regrouped, employ a different strategy, and get that train back on the tracks.

THE "END GAME"
At the end of the draft, whoever has the most money remaining can dictate how they want to fill out their roster. For example, if everyone else at the draft only has enough to bid $1/player, but your max is $4/player. You can say "$2" THREE times, and there is nothing anyone can do. You will win that player every time. Once everyone only has $1 remaining, the auction turns into a "snake draft" that goes round and round until each team has a full roster.

As you can see, the action and excitement of participating in an auction far outweigh your opportunities to grab the players you want over a snake draft. However, if you are looking to "take it to the next level," I can't speak highly enough about the auctions that the NFFC runs. The payouts, the competition, and most importantly, the lifelong friendships you will make are something you can't put a price on.

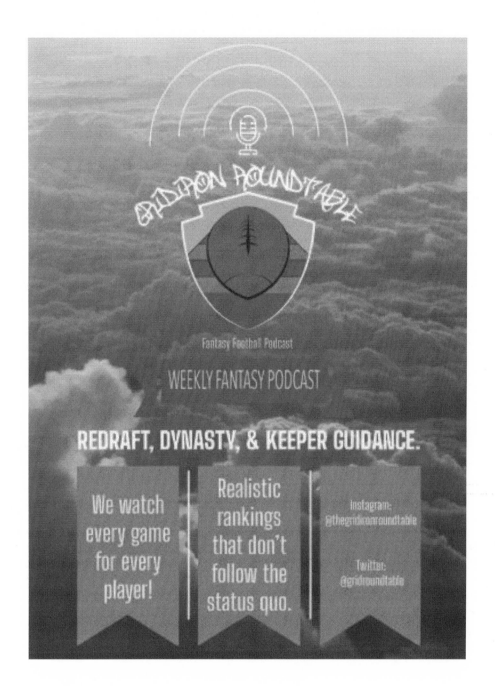

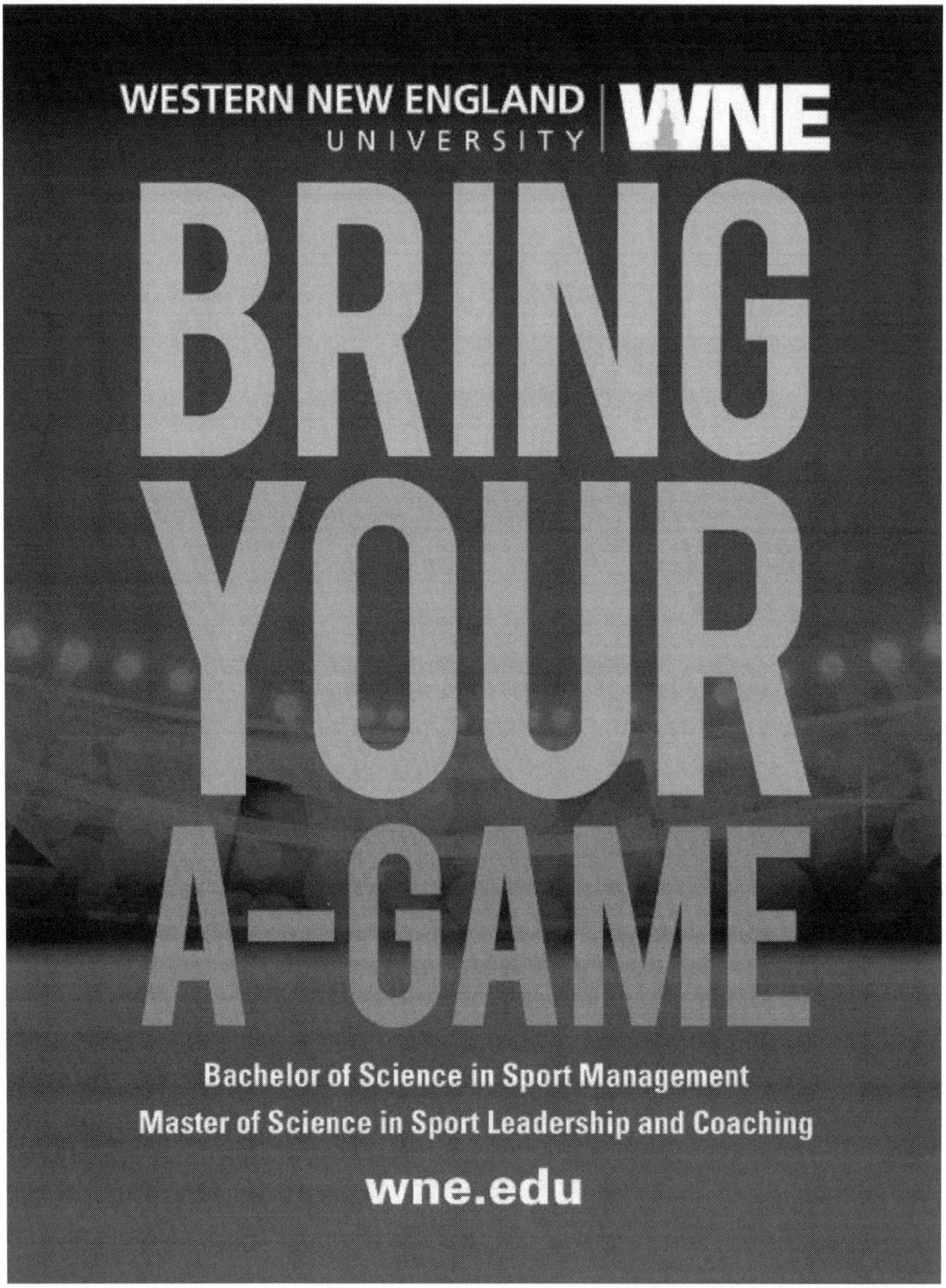

Chapter 3
OVERRATED AND UNDERRATED 2021

Every season, it's important to understand that just because a player is talented, that doesn't mean that they're necessarily worth the investment at their cost. Players coming off outlier great seasons, moving to bigger markets or even brand new to the league can oftentimes come with inflated costs in terms of draft capital. The inverse is also true. Steady players coming off an injury or down season, or aging veterans can be undervalued, making for a potentially excellent return on investment in drafts. My colleagues form The FantasyPros Fantasy Football Podcast (Mike Tagliere and Kyle Yates) were kind enough to join me for this quick roundtable discussion on players we think fit both of these categories in this year's upcoming fantasy football draft season.

OVERRATED

TAGS QB: AARON RODGERS GB - Rodgers played lights out in 2020, right? Not just touchdowns, but overall, he played like an MVP. If we were to simply dial back his touchdowns to his career rate of 6.3 percent (which is still elite – highest ever among quarterbacks with 3,800 career pass attempts), he would've finished as the QB10 last year. Him losing mobility in today's fantasy scene is bigger than most realize. Forget about the fact that he might not even play in 2021, he's overvalued.

YATES QB: JALEN HURTS PHI - Listen, Jalen Hurts has the potential to be a cheat code for fantasy football. With his rushing ability, there's a strong chance that he could give fantasy managers a safe floor each and every week he's on the field. However, buying into Hurts as a top-10 fantasy QB for 2021 is a very risky game to play. Just like Drew Lock in 2020, NFL defenses now have enough tape on Hurts where they're able to game plan on how to contain his rushing ability and make them beat him as a passer. With the receiving options he has at his disposal, there's a possibility that Hurts can do enough through the air to open things up in the run game, but that's too high of a cost for me to bet on that. As a result, there's a very good chance that Hurts' ADP spirals out of control this draft season.

JOE QB: JALEN HURTS PHI - Jalen Hurts has the potential to end up as a top 10 fantasy QB, but by no means is it necessary to draft him as such. You're passing over steady QB producers like Matt Ryan, Tom Brady, Matthew Stafford, and Ryan Tannehill when you do. Hurts is learning a new offense with a new HC/OC, and there are no guarantees that everything clicks for the Eagles offense right away. Everyone wants to be on the next big thing, but sometimes people ignore the downside. The offensive line didn't make enormous strides either. A Superflex reach, paired with a solid low-end QB1/high-end QB2, is a better risk than single QB leagues.

TAGS RB: ANTONIO GIBSON WAS - The average number of snaps played by top-12 running backs not named Antonio Gibson last year was 42.4 per game. Gibson himself averaged 28.9 snaps per game (no other running back averaged fewer than 34.2 snaps per game). Yes, Washington was trying to ease him into the running back role after he was utilized as a receiver in college, but it's still the same coaching staff in place, and J.D. McKissic is still there. On top of that, there is more surrounding talent, including Curtis Samuel, who's likely to get 20-plus carries himself. Ryan Fitzpatrick hasn't been one to check down throughout his career, so Gibson will need to score at an incredibly high rate if he wants to sniff low-end RB1/high-end RB2 numbers.

YATES RB: SAQUON BARKLEY NYG - From a talent perspective, Saquon Barkley is the best RB in the NFL when he's on the field. Unfortunately, the issue has been staying on the field the past two seasons. Barkley has played 15 out of a possible 32 games, making him a precarious investment at the top of your draft. For fantasy managers to have a shot of competing deep into their playoffs, they need their top draft pick to pull their weight all season long. As the RB3 in ECR right now, that's too high of a cost for Barkley that doesn't consider his injury history whatsoever. As a late first-round draft pick, the risk is worth the reward. A top-3 pick in your fantasy football draft might be a little bit too rich.

JOE RB: MILES SANDERS PHI - Miles Sanders has been released from Doug Pederson, but that doesn't make him a lock as an RB1. Currently, Sanders is hovering in that low-end RB1/high-end RB2 range and ahead of players coming off a better season (David Montgomery) or that have more upside (Najee Harris). Sanders is an explosive player, but so is his QB Jalen Hurts, who could steal some of those moments from Sanders in 2021. Oh, and why did they just bring in Kerryon Johnson too after drafting Kenneth Gainwell?

TAGS WR: KENNY GOLLADAY NYG- Golladay had the privilege of working with Matthew Stafford early in his NFL career, a quarterback who had no issues throwing into tight coverage, and no issues throwing the deep ball. While Daniel Jones isn't against throwing into tight coverage, he doesn't take many deep shots. The Giants suddenly have an extremely crowded room of pass catchers, as Golladay joins Sterling Shepard, Darius Slayton, Kadarius Toney, Evan Engram, Kyle Rudolph, and Saquon Barkley. It's just hard to see him getting 120-plus targets with all those viable options. When looking at receivers in the top-24, he gets me the least excited to roster.

YATES WR: MICHAEL THOMAS NO - Michael Thomas has been among the fantasy elite the past couple of seasons (minus 2020), but that was when Drew Brees was his QB. With Brees' propensity to get the ball out quickly underneath, Thomas was force-fed the ball, and he became the consensus WR1 in all of fantasy football last year because of it. With that being said, Brees is no longer playing in the NFL, and Thomas has some uncertainty at QB. Things could be great for Thomas if James Winston is his QB, or they could be a little rough with Taysom Hill as the full-time starter. With this amount of risk in place, it's hard to justify Thomas' ranking in the top-10 of FantasyPros' ECR right now. He could finish within the top-5 when it's all said and done - or he could finish outside the top-30. That's too much risk for me at this point of the off-season. *(Update: Thomas likely missing at least first month of season knocks his value down further)*

JOE WR: KENNY GOLLADAY NYG - I love Kenny Golladay as a talent, and he's getting a lot of attention because he signed in New York — perhaps too much attention. Daniel Jones is a turnover machine during his tenure with the Giants, and it's difficult for a fantasy wide receiver to excel when his QB takes the ball out of his hands. The downgrade from Matthew Stafford to Daniel Jones is significant, and Golladay draws some tough CB opponents to open the season. The 'too big to fail' theory didn't play out well in Denver last year. Don't chase it again in New York.

TAGS TE: IRV SMITH MIN - We've been saying, "just wait until the Vikings get rid of Kyle Rudolph." That was when we were supposed to see Smith's breakout. Well, unfortunately for him, Justin Jefferson came around. Despite the Vikings inflating their pass attempts last year, the combination of Rudolph and Smith netted just 80 targets. Even if Smith received all of Rudolph's departed targets, that's no guarantee to net top-12 production. Their defense should get back on track this year, and it's not like Jefferson will become less involved. You shouldn't be paying for top-12 production, but rather hoping for it.

YATES TE: KYLE PITTS ATL - Kyle Pitts has the potential to be truly special for fantasy football. Within a year or two, it would not surprise me at all if we're talking about Pitts as the consensus TE1 off the board. For his rookie season, though, it's hard to get behind a top-8 ranking already at this point. It's highly likely that we see that number rise even further by the time drafts start happening, which means that I will have zero shares of Pitts in my leagues. For him to return that value, he has to put up one of the best seasons for a rookie TE we've ever seen, which is too much for me to bet on. Can he do it? Absolutely. Do I want to put all my chips in on that happening? Absolutely not.

JOE TE: GEORGE KITTLE SF: Tags will HATE me for this one, and I am a huge George Kittle fan. He's absolutely a top-tier TE, but I don't want to pay heavy draft capital for a tight end not named Travis Kelce. Kittle is surrounded by far better WR talent than when he had his 2018 breakout of 1,300 yards. He's also never had more than 5 TD's in a season. If the narrative is Jimmy Garoppolo will struggle and Trey lance takes over, how do those struggles affect Kittle's production? And does Trey Lance immediately become the "cure-all"? The uncertainty means, at his ADP, I would instead be drafting RBs, WR2's or elite QB talent, which is basically what his draft range is.

UNDERRATED

TAGS QB: LAMAR JACKSON BAL - Why is Jackson falling in drafts? His current ranking in the community is QB4. Over the last two years, Jackson has scored 748.5 fantasy points while no other quarterback has topped 689.3 fantasy points. The Ravens actually gave him support at wide receiver this offseason, bringing in Rashod Bateman, Sammy Watkins, and Tylan Wallace, yet he's going to be less valuable? We aren't even close to the point where we have to start worrying about Jackson's rushing upside fading, either.

YATES QB: CAM NEWTON NE - Do I want to tie myself completely to Cam Newton for the entire 2021 season? Absolutely not. However, a healthy Cam Newton can still do phenomenal things for fantasy football. To start the season, Newton should get off to a hot start and he now has the receiving weapons around him to make life easier. With the rushing upside - particularly his use around the goal line - Newton's a fantastic late-round QB target. As long as he's fully healthy, Newton will be a safe start in fantasy leagues this year.

JOE QB: KIRK COUSINS MIN - In September of 2019, Cousins threw for just 3 TDs and 2 INT with 183 passing YPG. For the next two months, Cousins threw for 18 TDs and 1 INT with 288 passing YPG. Through Cousins' first six games of 2020, 11 TD/10 INT/245 passing YPG. Over the next ten games, 24 TD/3 INT/279 passing YPG. One year is an anomaly. Two years is a trend. Cousins may never be a perfect QB in fantasy or reality, but when he's on a good run, he's a QB1.

TAGS RB: NAJJE HARRIS PIT - Running backs are at their prime when they enter the NFL, which makes them the most valuable their rookie season, unlike quarterbacks, wide receivers, and tight ends. Because of that, Harris, who takes over as the Steelers' lead back, is someone you want to have on your roster. The Steelers are a team that hasn't been shy about giving running backs 18-plus touches per game with Mike Tomlin at the helm. You don't draft a three-down back like Harris in the first round and put him in some timeshare. I wouldn't be surprised to see him average 20-plus touches per game, which puts him smack dab in the middle of the RB1 conversation.

YATES RB: TARIK COHEN CHI - Let's go a little bit further down the board for this player, shall we? Tarik Cohen is coming back from a season-ending injury in 2021, but his price tag right now is too good to not at least highlight. Ranked in the RB40's over at FantasyPros' ECR, Cohen is going to be too involved in this offense to not return that value. With a limited QB in Andy Dalton to start the season, Cohen should be targeted heavily out of the backfield as a receiver. If Cohen gets off to a hot start this season, look to flip him for peak value before Justin Fields takes over and capitalize on the return on investment.

JOE RB: TRAVIS ETIENNE JAC - Travis Etienne is being drafted right at the end of RB2/top of RB3 but I think his impact will be far greater. James Robinson was a great story and league winner in 2020, but as an undrafted FA from another regime, I doubt his presence will slow down the inevitable rise of Travis Etienne with the Jags. First round draft capital spent on an RB is rare nowadays, and his built-in relationship with Trevor Lawrence is not to be underestimated. As the year goes on, he will get stronger as a potential low end RB1 finisher.

TAG WR: JULIO JONES TEN - There are too many people writing Jones off after an injury-plagued 2020 season. Don't say he's injury prone. He played at least 14 games in each of the previous six seasons. Even better? His performance didn't decline in 2020, as the 11.3 yards per target he averaged was a career-high. He played just nine games, but he was on pace for 91 receptions, 1,371 yards, and six touchdowns, which would've been right in line with his previous seasons. Getting him as a WR2 is theft.

YATES WR: ROBERT WOODS LAR - Even with a mid-range WR2 price tag in FantasyPros' ECR, Robert Woods might be flying under the radar a bit. Woods has finished above that mark each of the past three seasons and he now gets a major upgrade at QB. Matthew Stafford is going to unlock a whole other side of this playbook that Sean McVay hasn't been able to utilize yet and Woods could stand to benefit in a big way. Last season, Woods was on nearly every one of my fantasy rosters. If his price tag stays the same as it is right now, it'll be the same thing again for 2021.

JOE WR: CEEDEE LAMB DAL - CeeDee Lamb had 74 rec on 111 targets for 936 yards with 7 TDs as a rookie. Justin Jefferson's incredible rookie campaign overshadowed Lamb's outstanding first year effort. The fact that Lamb only played 4.5 games with Dak Prescott and still put up those stats speaks to just how good he could be in '21. He's being drafted around WR20, but he has a real shot to finish as a top 10 WR this year.

TAGS TE: TYLER HIGBEE LAR - The per-play production out of Higbee has been consistent over the last three years in Sean McVay's offense. Notice how I didn't say per-game production? His yards per target have remained steady in-between 8.2 and 8.7, so all you really need is the volume. The departure of Gerald Everett creates a massive opportunity for Higbee, and we saw what that can look like at the end of the 2019 season when Everett was hurt, and Higbee racked up 43 receptions for 522 yards and two touchdowns over a five-game span. Now with Matthew Stafford under center, Higbee should come with a top-six ceiling.

YATES TE: JONNU SMITH NE - For anyone that follows my work, you know the name that I'm about to mention. Jonnu Smith received a big contract from New England in the off-season and the Patriots clearly have a need for him in this offense. Hunter Henry's presence on this roster will keep Jonnu's ADP down, but he has the talent to smash that cost investment. The Patriots clearly have a plan for him in this system and he should be force fed the ball. Outside the top-12 at the TE position gets pretty gross quickly, but Smith's going to be a must-add option if he stays in this range.

JOE TE: JONNU SMITH NE - I can't believe how much I agree with Yates in this section, but he's dead on when it comes to Jonnu Smith. I've been leading this charge all off season that the Pats targeted Smith to make him the focal point of the offense and whether it's Cam Newton (who had a nice run with Greg Olsen), or Mac Jones (young QB's love checking down to those TEs), Smith should be in a very stable place. Hunter Henry is NOT a deterrent for me at all when it comes to drafting Smith. In fact, it wouldn't surprise me if Smith outscored Kyle Pitts in 2021, who will be drafted rounds before. We have yet to scratch the surface of how good Smith can be, and the Pats' brain trust knows how to use a talented TE talent when they have it.

Chapter 4

QUARTERBACKS

Joe Pisapia

	SINGLE QB LEAGUE			QB2 SUPERFLEX	
	Player	RPV		Player	RPV
1	Patrick Mahomes II	10%	1	Joe Burrow	14%
2	Josh Allen	9%	2	Jalen Hurts	14%
3	Kyler Murray	7%	3	Kirk Cousins	13%
4	Lamar Jackson	6%	4	Deshaun Watson *	6%
5	Dak Prescott	4%	5	Trevor Lawrence	2%
6	Russell Wilson	0%	6	Ben Roethlisberger	-1%
7	Aaron Rodgers	0%	7	Baker Mayfield	-1%
8	Ryan Tannehill	-1%	8	Derek Carr	-3%
9	Justin Herbert	-7%	9	Ryan Fitzpatrick	-3%
10	Tom Brady	-9%	10	Tua Tagavailoa	-9%
11	Matthew Stafford	-9%	11	Carson Wentz	-12%
12	Matt Ryan	-11%	12	Jared Goff	-19%

****See Page 3 for information on how to get RPV Cheat Sheets for one-time fee with free updates in July and August after one time purchase***

OVERVIEW

In last year's quarterback overview, I wrote a mini-manifesto advising people to change their QB approach in single QB leagues. Yes, talent is abundant in the position. However, the top dogs are separating from the elite range to SUPER-elite. Three years ago, Patrick Mahomes emerged, followed by Lamar Jackson, then Kyler Murray and Josh Allen last season. Oh, and Dak Prescott was on a crazy pace before his injury Week 5. The QB revolution is here! It's also young and NFL-ready more than ever. To put it simply, the league is set up for quarterbacks to excel by protecting them. Plus, the young QBs are more familiar with pro-style offenses in their college days. Moving to a 17-game season only exacerbates all of these facts.

The top 5 QBs are indeed a distinct cut above the rest. After that, you have to deal with some questions: the regression year over year of Aaron Rodgers, Russell Wilson's unhappiness with the Seahawks, the repeatability question of Justin Herbert, the age of Tom Brady, Matt Ryan, and Matthew Stafford, and the walking question mark that is Deshaun Watson right now. The good news is that QB2 is flush with upside like Jalen Hurts, Carson Wentz, and of course, Joe Burrow. Not to mention Trevor Lawrence and a rookie class that could see the field relatively quickly in 2021.

In Superflex, I would still make every attempt to add two QB1's to your roster and up your RPV advantage over other teams. Although QB2 has an upside, stability can be uncertain. I would not be afraid to draft Trey Lance, Justin Fields, or Zack Wilson as my third QB for bye weeks/second half of the season. Some boring veterans like Kirk Cousins, Ben Roethlisberger, and Derek Carr can also get the job done at QB2 if you miss out on that second run in a draft.

THE ELITE

1. **Patrick Mahomes, KC:** There may be some annual contenders for the overall QB point leader. However, Patrick Mahomes will annually be in the top tier, which keeps him the #1 overall QB. In 2020, Mahomes threw for 4.7K yards and 38 TD in 15 games. It's hard to find a flaw in his game, and weekly he does something we've never seen before at the position. He has a HOF coach, the #1 TE in the game, and a top WR. He also has every intangible you could ask for in a quarterback. It's scary to think how good he could be when all is said and done. He continues to limit mistakes (6 INT in '20, 5 INT in '19), and with 17 games next season, he could realistically make another run at 5K passing yards. He went over 25 fantasy points in seven games last season and over 30 points five times, all but winning you those weeks if you rostered him. The question is: when to take Mahomes? In a shallow single QB league (10 teams), you'd think you would pass on him. However, I would advise the opposite. The top 10 QBs on the board are robust. Therefore, Mahomes could prove to be an essential advantage. In a 12-team single QB league, you can make a case for as early as the turn in a snake draft rounds 2-3. The WR pool is bottomless, and you can make up ground there. You can fade Mahomes with a powerful QB1 class this year if you like, but there may not be a better one than Mahomes in terms of quality investment. In Superflex leagues, he's easily a top 5 overall selection.

2. **Josh Allen, BUF:** Here's a selection from what I wrote about Josh Allen in the 2018 Fantasy Football Black Book: *"In terms of raw QB talent, (Josh) Allen could be a game-changer...Allen has the highest ceiling of any QB in this ('18) draft class, in my opinion."* In that same profile, I wrote about how imperative it was to surround Allen with excellent WR options and refine his mechanics. After 2020, we can safely check both of those boxes, as Allen went onto have an MVP caliber season and a finish as QB1 overall in fantasy. He finished '20 with 4.5K passing yards, a 69% completion rate, 37 TD, and 10 INT. His rushing attempts year over year stayed flat, but his yardage fell from 510 to 421 yards. That's probably a good thing because it meant he wasn't running with abandon as much. However, he still managed eight rush TDs. Outside of one dreadful game in Week 7 vs. SEA, the O-Line played well, but the run game made the Bills one-dimensional offensively, and Allen to Stefon Diggs was pretty much that dimension. In the playoffs, "reckless" Josh Allen started to creep back in as he tried to do too much under pressure, twisting and turning, trying to make plays instead of eating a sack or throwing a ball away. More balance from the run game in 2021 will help the Bills and Allen thrive this season. However, that's not a given. Six times, Josh Allen scored 30+ fantasy points. A fantasy regular season is usually 13-14 weeks long. He's good for six wins, and that puts you in the playoff hunt.

3. **Kyler Murray, ARZ:** At the mid-point of last season, Kyler Murray was on pace to make history as the first QB to ever rush for 1K yards and pass for 4K. He closed the season at 3,971 passing yards and 819 rushing yards. This was due in part to being crushed Week 11 and tweaking his shoulder. The next few weeks, Murray did his best, but he was not 100% healthy. That's the risk/reward of Kyler Murray. At 5'10" and 207 lbs, he doesn't have the same size as Josh Allen, but he plays the same style. It's why I would recommend backing up any investment in him with a solid QB2 on your bench as an insurance policy, even in a single QB league. D'Andre Hopkins was a considerable addition last year, and the two developed fantastic chemistry right away. The inconsistency of the run game and the play-calling created some drastic swings in the offense's productivity. A 4K/1K yard season is certainly within his grasp in 2021, as are 10+ rushing TDs (Murray was 2nd among all QBs with 11 in '20). Last year was a preview of how special Murray can be. Let's hope that Kliff Kingsbury and poor health don't screw it all up again.

4. **Dak Prescott, DAL:** Through the first four weeks of the season, Dak Prescott led all QB's in fantasy points with 125. That incredible start was due in part to an abundance of top-level offensive weapons, coupled with a dreadful defense incapable of holding any lead. The good news is the defense has not markedly improved year over year, and the offensive weapons are all returning. Prescott's brutal ankle injury was undoubtedly a backbreaker for many fantasy players, but all reports on his recovery have been solid, and he's always been a hard worker. Dak's phenomenal 2020 start should have been no surprise considering he fell just shy of 5K passing yards in 2019. I fully expect him to challenge that level again in 2021, with 30+ TDs. If he does, you have an elite fantasy QB on your roster at a slightly lower ADP than the top tier.

That's the perfect storm in single QB leagues. In Superflex, Dak is a first-round talent. There's a strong possibility he finishes as QB1 overall in 2021.

5. **Lamar Jackson, BAL:** It would have been impossible for Lamar Jackson to duplicate his lofty 2019 performance of 420 fantasy points. For the first 11 weeks, it seemed like a combination of the league catching up to the Ravens' scheme and the Ravens being cautious with their best weapon. What resulted were lackluster results. After a Week 12 absence, Jackson posted 80 or more rushing yards in 4 of his last five games, where he finished as a QB1 in each of those final five contests. The Ravens have not given Lamar Jackson a true #1 wide receiver. Hollywood Brown and Sammy Watkins do NOT qualify as such. The force-feeding of Mark Andrews was a separate issue early on, and if the Ravens are going to have success, they simply must continue to be a heavy "run first" team. We will see if Rashod Bateman can develop quickly, but you can't necessarily count on that right away. Jackson was a better pocket passer in college than one may think. The trouble comes back to this team not having a WR who can separate, and the offensive line is built for the run game, not pass protection. Despite relative disappointment compared to lofty expectations, Jackson still finished as QB 10 overall. Had he played one more game, he may have realistically finished top 5. A more confident Lamar Jackson, coming off exercising playoff demons, is one you should be aggressive on in 2021. After all, it is only his fourth year in the league, and he's still an elite fantasy QB.

TOP TALENT

1. **Russell Wilson, SEA:** The MVP narrative was rolling along for the first nine weeks of the season for Russell Wilson, as he averaged 29.5 pts per game. After that, Wilson averaged just 17.5 pts the rest of the way, killing his MVP candidacy and many fantasy playoff hopes as well. Wilson is a steady presence, despite the down ending in 2020. He should be a lock for 4+K yards and around 35 TDs. The notion the Seahawks were shopping him seriously this offseason is laughable. The franchise QB isn't going anywhere. Last season, Wilson's rushing yards went back above the 500 mark, and his 42 combined passing and rushing TDs were a career-high. At 32, Wilson is in his prime and is an excellent redraft or dynasty investment. D.K. Metcalf's emerging star, coupled with the familiarity of Tyler Lockett, a returning Chris Carson, and an exciting slot WR option drafted in D'Wayne Eskridge, should keep Wilson high on the fantasy QB scale again at season's end. He could be the best return on investment in the position.

2. **Justin Herbert, LAC:** Justin Herbert was a huge miss collectively by the fantasy community at large. No one thought he would be that good, and if they did, no one thought he would be that good that quickly. Herbert set a rookie record for passing TDs (31), threw just ten picks, and crossed 4.3K yards on his way to Rookie of the Year honors. A new coaching staff, including a new OC, should be careful not to screw up a good thing. The new OC is Joe Lombardi, former QB coach of the Saints. Learning under Sean Payton and Drew Brees, expectations are high for Herbert and company. The expectations are a more "up-tempo" offense built around Herbert's strengths. Drafting Rashawn Slater goes a long way to helping improve an offensive line that struggled. With (8) 300-yard games, Herbert had some big days in 2020, but he also had some rookie moments. Suppose you draft Herbert, bid on a similar season to 2020, not necessarily upside for more. He's not as safe as some veterans like Russell Wilson, nor do I think he has the upside in startup dynasty leagues like Trevor Lawrence or Joe Burrow. But the 23-year-old QB was impressive enough year one to consider him a QB1 in 2021.

SOLID OPTIONS

1. **Aaron Rodgers, GB:** I know Aaron Rodgers had an elite level season, but at 38 this year, it's better to think of him as just a hair behind that top 5 group. He threw for a league-high 48 TDs and just five picks while posting 4,299 yards passing and 387 fantasy points. Everything broke right for Rodgers in 2020. Well, except for the NFC Championship game. Oh, and the fact he's "disgruntled" with the organization. It's important not to lose sight of the fact that Rodgers threw for 25 TDs in '18 and 26 TDs in '19. The 48

seems like a pretty colossal outlier at this stage in his career. He had a three-week period where he threw for 15 TDs. Rodgers will give you consistently solid QB play and is still a reliable, upper-tier QB in fantasy. It would be foolish to bid on 2020 as though it was repeatable. Davante Adams had a lot to do with Rodgers' success. If Adams should suffer any injury again, Rodgers' value would immediately take a massive hit. This is the significant difference between Rodgers and a QB like Matt Ryan, who has more weapons at his disposal. For the second year in a row, Green Bay failed to bring in a complementary WR of note, although bringing back Aaron Jones is beneficial to the offense.

2. **Tom Brady, TB:** The entire regular season was one giant practice session for Tom Brady and the Bucs to get right for the playoffs. Not only did they click at the right time, but they went on to win a Super Bowl (Tom Brady's 7th title and 10th appearance). He was supposed to slow down, fade away, etc. It's not happening. Just accept it. Brady has his gang coming back again for '21. A healthy Chris Godwin will be scary, along with Mike Evans and Antonio Brown, over an entire season. The most critical return may be running back Leonard Fournette. In these last few years of Brady's career, he's been at his best running play action effectively. Fournette's emergence late in the year carried over into the playoffs, was a big part of the Bucs' run in the playoffs. Five of his last seven regular-season games went over 340+ passing yards. It's hard not to see Brady realistically approaching 4.5K yards and 30+ TDs again in '21. Brady finished as QB8 overall, and he should be drafted as a QB1 this season again in fantasy. We should all find something in life we love as much as Tom Brady loves to play football and prove people wrong.

3. **Matthew Stafford, LAR:** Matthew Stafford deserves some wins. For 12 years, Stafford has toiled away with mostly awful Lions teams. Now, he goes to sunny Los Angeles with a boy wonder offensive coach. He also brings a creaky back and a recently operated on thumb, but Stafford finds himself in a unique situation. He has a second act to show everyone how underrated he indeed has been for the last decade. Since 2011, Stafford has thrown for 4K yards 8 times. One would think he should be a lock for that in '21 as long as health cooperates. Unfortunately, the Rams gave up Jared Goff, a '21 3rd round pick, and their 1st rounders in '22 & '23. If this experiment fails, the Rams could implode quickly, considering their cap issues and lack of early draft picks the next two seasons. However, I'm inclined to think Stafford will find new life with Sean McVay and this talented offense. As a result, Stafford should be considered a low-end QB1 in fantasy this season.

4. **Matt Ryan, ATL:** I, for one, am excited to see what Arthur Smith and his staff do with this Falcons team. Smith did a great job with the Titans' offense as their coordinator. He's not bringing Derrick Henry with him, so expect the Falcons' offensive strength to still be the passing game. Matt Ryan had two elite wide receivers in Julio Jones and Calvin Ridley, but Julio is now onto Tennessee. The addition of TE sensation Kyle Pitts in the draft could fill that void and running back Mike Davis in free agency gives Ryan a complete and balanced complement of weapons. Ryan is an annual threat to throw for 4.5K yards and close to 30 TDs. The Falcons still didn't make any real gains year over year defensively, so this offense will have plenty of opportunities to put up points. That's good for your fantasy team. Ryan is a "safe" consolation prize at QB if you miss out on the upper tier at the position.

HIGHS AND LOWS

1. **Ryan Tannehill, TEN:** 2020 was a roller coaster for the Titans and QB Ryan Tannehill. The fact he finished as a QB1 (8) times and a QB2 (8) times says it all. He finished with 3.8K yards, 33 passing TDs, and seven rushing TDs. Ideally, you want Tannehill as your second QB in a Superflex format. That bonus upside he brings some weeks can be huge. However, as your starting quarterback in a single QB format, the inconsistencies could hurt you some weeks. The Titans lost Corey Davis and Jonnu Smith to free agency, but added Julio Jones in June to create one of the more formidable WR corps in the NFL. Tannehill has established himself as a fantasy-worthy QB, it's just that no one seems to give him his due. The Jones addition will raise that profile, but overpaying for Tannehill isn't advisable either. He's a lower end QB1.

2. **Joe Burrow, CIN:** Before the ACL tear, Joe Burrow looked very much like an emerging star at QB for the Bengals. He was on pace for 4.3K yards and around 25 combined TDs. In the good news department, the Bengals drafted his favorite target Ja'Marr Chase from LSU to add to an already strong WR group, Tee Higgins and Tyler Boyd. They did pick up two offensive linemen, Jackson Carman and D'Ante Smith, as

well. They had both better perform because Burrow was sacked 31 times in 10 weeks (2nd most sacks taken by a QB in '20). But the best news, besides the fact Joe Burrow is medically on track for the start of the season, is that the Bengals defense is still going to be deficient in 2021. That means Joe Burrow will constantly be looking to put up points, and that's fantasy gold. He threw for 300 yards in 5 of his ten games last season and should be well over 4K yards in 2021. The one caveat here is that although Burrow was sneaky mobile in college, you may see a more conservative approach for him post major knee surgery. Burrow is a top 10 dynasty QB, and in 2021, he should be considered a low-endQB1. Just know, there will be some highs and lows in that game log. You need a consistent roster around him if you have playoff aspirations.

WILD CARDS

1. **Jalen Hurts, PHI:** Let me say I am a fan of Jalen Hurts, the quarterback. He bet on himself in college and won, then showed he could play at the NFL level in 2020. I am not, however, completely sold on Jalen Hurts, the fantasy quarterback, quite yet. His 38-point performance against the Cardinals rightfully excited a lot of fantasy analysts. But there were some less than stellar moments as well that folks are forgetting. His rushing upside is incredibly intriguing, but he still has a long way to go as a passer. People are also ignoring the Eagles offensive line that did not get markedly better year over year. Plus, it's a new HC, and that means a new playbook to learn and execute. I am not saying Hurts can't take his new toy DeVonta Smith and have himself a QB1 season. I am saying the risk of him finishing outside of the QB1 range is equally possible. Therefore, drafting ahead of proven entities like Tom Brady, Matt Ryan, etc., is unnecessary in a single QB format. In a Superflex league, the gamble becomes intriguing because you can easily team him up with one of those steadier veterans and enjoy the high ceiling games without the low floor contests costing you weeks. In dynasty leagues, Hurts needs to show himself to be the QB of the future for the Eagles, or Nick Sirianni may get to choose his guy in the 2022 draft. In my opinion, the best place to have shares of Hurts in 2021 is best-ball and DFS.
2. **Baker Mayfield, CLE:** Baker Mayfield has had some challenges in his first three seasons; different HC and play-callers every year, injuries around him, and lofty expectations. In the second half of last season, Nick Chubb got healthy, the offense got simplified, and Mayfield became very proficient in running lots of play-action, forcing him to be more direct with the football. This was the secret to the Browns' success last year. A less reckless Baker Mayfield was a better quarterback in 2020. The throws you get away with in college are interceptions in the NFL. Ironically, this "Better Baker" evolved with Odell Beckham Jr. on the shelf. He will continue to have some decent moments, but in reality, he's a QB2 in Superflex who will have plenty of all or nothing weeks. If he can pick up where he left off (14 TD/2 INT over his last eight games to close out 2020), he could sneak into the back end of QB1. But even over that good second half, Mayfield put up 31 fantasy points against the Ravens and just 8 points against the 2-win Jets. Mayfield is an inconsistent asset until proven otherwise over an entire season. It is also fair to remember two of his home games last year were in weather conditions that made throwing the football nearly impossible.
3. **Carson Wentz, IND:** In 2017, Carson Wentz threw 33 TDs in 13 games before blowing out his knee. When he returned for 11 games in 2018, he threw for 21 TD. In 2018, Wentz played all 16 games, threw for 4K yards and 27 TDs. Here's what I am getting at: I know last year was an unmitigated disaster for Wentz, but that offensive line was atrocious. Like Philp Rivers before him, Wentz is going from one of the worst offensive lines in football to the Colts (one of the best). Rivers settled in nicely eventually and led the Colts to the playoffs and nearly an upset of the Bills on the road in the playoffs. Now, throw in the fact some of those strong seasons I mentioned at the top were with Frank Reich, the present coach of the Colts. When coach and QB speak the same language, it's infinitely easier to get off on the right foot in a new situation. I am not ready to throw away Wentz, and he's a great buy low in Superflex dynasty formats. In redraft Superflex leagues, he could be an excellent value. The offense is balanced, and just getting away from the Philadelphia media blitz will go a long way for Wentz's psyche. If all breaks right, Wentz can be a top 15 QB this season at a discounted cost. ***UPDATE: A foot injury could cause Wentz to miss the start of the season impacting his Superflex value a great deal. Monitor that situation closely.***

VETERAN PRESENCE

1. **Kirk Cousins, MIN:** I'm going to make an unpopular statement: Kirk Cousins is a better fantasy quarterback than you realize. He's just a slow starter. I will now elaborate. In September of 2019, Cousins threw for just 3 TDs and 2 INT with 183 passing YPG. For the next two months, Cousins threw for 18 TDs and 1 INT with 288 passing YPG. Through Cousins' first six games of 2020, 11 TD/10 INT/245 passing YPG. Over the next ten games, 24 TD/3 INT/279 passing YPG. One year is an anomaly. Two years is a trend. Cousins may never be a perfect QB in fantasy or reality, but when he's on a good run, he's a QB1. He finished as such in 6 of his eight last games to close out the season. Those runs make him very appealing in DFS at specific points, as he will be undervalued. As your second QB in Superflex, he is a strong option. As a QB1 in deeper leagues, you'd like a tad more consistency, but Cousins has an excellent complement of weapons and is still just 32 years old. Expect 4k yards and 30 TDs in 2021, just be prepared for a slow start, which by the way, could make Cousins an excellent trade target in October.

2. **Ben Roethlisberger, PIT:** A more balanced offense would be good for Ben Roethlisberger's fantasy value. The Steelers' ineptitude running the football made the offense far too predictable. Big Ben went from low-end QB1 during their undefeated start to a low-end QB2 during their collapse. At 39, injury is always a risk, but as a Superflex QB2, he's safe in terms of value on the board. He has three talented wide receivers, a new star RB in Najee Harris from Alabama, and a talented young TE from Penn State named Pat Freiermuth (although rookie TE's tend not to deliver early). The offensive line is still not great, limiting his upside in matchups against teams with an intense pass rush. Roethlisberger and the Steelers' attack will continue to be less aggressive than years passed. For clarity, Big Ben averaged just 6.3 yards per attempt. That was worse than Drew Lock and Mitchell Trubisky towards the very bottom of the league. He's serviceable at this point as a QB2 but lacks the weekly upside of his younger peers.

3. **Ryan Fitzpatrick, WAS:** The bearded one can still sling the rock. Last season, Ryan Fitzpatrick averaged 8.3 yards per attempt and got the Dolphins off to a solid start before being replaced by the "QB of the Future," Tua Tagovailoa. Despite a forgettable Week 1 performance, Fitzpatrick turned in 5 straight 21+ point performances before getting the hook in a blowout against the Jets in Week 6. You can't blame the Dolphins, but the move may have indeed cost them the playoffs in 2020. Now, Fitzmagic gets another opportunity to play in his first playoff game, but for the Washington Football Team. He inherits a pretty solid complement of weapons across the board and some great matchups against some soft NFC East defenses. Fitz will be an excellent streaming QB in 2021 and a decent Superflex starter most weeks. Officially, Washington says he's "competing" for the starting job, but it's his. Despite imperfections, Washington had upgraded year over year from a genuinely awful quarterback carousel in 2020.

4. **Derek Carr, LV:** Very quietly, Derek Carr finished as QB13 last season. This was due to him playing in all 16 games, which many QBs did not in 2020. Carr did throw for his 3rd straight 4k yard season, but I have significant concerns about the offensive line turnover for the Raiders. At 30, Derek Carr is a prototypical league-average quarterback, hence the 8-8 record of the Raiders. I would love him as my 3rd QB in Superflex, but starting him more than twice a year isn't the best plan. Although Carr did make some statistical strides, it's hard to get excited about him in fantasy terms.

REDEMPTION SONGS

1. **Tua Tagovailoa, MIA:** I understand Tua Tagovailoa's debut was not stellar in 2020. Between significant hip surgery, no OTA's, no preseason, and a QB controversy in his locker room, it's a wonder he could do anything productive on the field. However, the Dolphins continued to build the right way and added WR Will Fuller on a one-year "show me" deal and WR Jaylen Waddle via the draft. Tua has the weapons and an entire offseason to reach his potential in 2021. He's a ferocious competitor and an intelligent QB. He just needs some time to get his feet under him. In 9 starts, he threw for just 11 TDs, but the new weapons

will open up the field more for the young QB. He remains a perfect buy low in Superflex dynasty leagues. In redraft formats, he could be a decent mid-range QB2. Tua's bottom line is a work in progress but one that still carries more potential than some want to acknowledge.

2. **Sam Darnold, CAR:** I am cautiously optimistic that the bulk of Sam Darnold's NFL failure can be attributed to Adam Gase. Not all of it, but enough of a chunk that I am buying into the Darnold reclamation project the Panthers have taken on in 2021. He goes from being bereft of weapons to having arguably the best RB in football in Christian McCaffrey and two talented receivers in DJ Moore and Robby Anderson (whom Darnold is familiar with from their Jet days). He will also benefit from OC Joe Brady, whom I thought was one of the top play-callers in the NFL last year, and stunned he didn't receive more attention as an HC candidate around the league. Three years ago, Darnold was an excellent QB prospect. At 23 years old, it's far too soon to throw him away. It remains to be seen if he can become a fantasy asset, but as your 3rd QB in a Superflex, man, I would love to have him on some rosters to find out.

SWAN SONGS

1. **Jared Goff, DET:** Jared Goff was not the same dude without peak Todd Gurley in that Rams offense. Even during those days, Goff made plenty of head-shaking decisions, and Sean McVay simply had enough. Now, Goff has been banished to Detroit into a team rebuilding, yet again. The weapons are below average, but the offensive line graded out at 12th overall in PFF and added Penei Sewell in the draft. Still, it's hard not to imagine Goff will be toiling away in Detroit and become fantasy irrelevant for the remainder of his career. As a 3rd QB in a Superflex for bye weeks is the only viable reason to roster Goff.

2. **Jimmy Garoppolo, SF:** Yes, the 49ers made a Super Bowl with Jimmy Garoppolo. The 49ers also just moved heaven and earth to get Trey Lance on their roster. Garoppolo has made just 25 starts for San Francisco over the last few years. He has a cumbersome contract and struggles to throw the ball downfield. He's also not the athlete Trey Lance is, and it would be shocking for Lance to sit an entire season under Jimmy G, effectively missing two straight seasons on the field (the other due to Lance sitting out 2020 during the pandemic). There's an outside chance Garoppolo plays in fewer games this season for the 49ers than Lance. He's simply not a good fantasy investment in the current environment surrounding him, and frankly, even when he's been on the field, he hasn't dazzled enough to get excited about.

3. **Cam Newton, NE:** Cam Newton finished as QB16 last year despite showing zero aptitude for the Patriots passing scheme. Granted, the Patriots' lack of weapons did not make it easy for Newton to succeed. In 15 games, Newton threw for just 2,657 yards, 8 TDs, and 10 INTs. However, it was his 12 rushing TDs that saved his fantasy bacon. Will that be enough for Newton on a one-year deal with the Pats to hold off Mac Jones? Unfortunately, I think the answer is no. Even though I love the Jonnu Smith signing, the additions of Nelson Agholor, Kendrick Bourne, and Hunter Henry don't exactly strike fear into the hearts of opposing defenses. With an accurate attack, though, they could be a proficient group. Unfortunately, that's where Cam particularly struggles and where Mac Jones could potentially shine. As a result, the prospects of Newton playing 17 games at QB for the Pats this year are slim, which makes him a lousy fantasy asset.

4. **Daniel Jones, NYG:** Daniel Jones is a turnover machine. In the 27 NFL games he's played in, Jones has 29 fumbles and 22 INTs. The one crutch is that when Saquon Barkley is healthy, he's been a better version of himself statistically. A healthy run game goes a long way for any QB, but Wayne Gallman had some strong games last year, while Jones continued to spiral. The Giants offensive line is still nothing to write home about. The curious mish-mosh of WR receiver additions year over year (Kenny Golladay, John Ross, Kadarius Toney) have set Jones up for a situation where it all doesn't come together, the Giants (and all of their massive 2022 draft capital) will be selecting another QB. Last year, the Broncos created a similar situation surrounding QB Drew Lock with so much talent it appeared "too big to fail," but it failed nonetheless. This may be the end for Daniel Jones.

5. **Teddy Bridgewater/Drew Lock, DEN:** I would give Teddy Bridgewater the early lead in the starting QB sweepstakes for the Broncos simply because they traded picks for him. Teddy was serviceable last year at times but didn't light up the stat sheet. The Denver offense is loaded with talent. It's all about whether they can stay healthy. Javonte Williams could help this backfield led by Melvin Gordon (for now) and take

pressure off whoever is under center to find Courtland Sutton, Jerry Jeudy, Noah Fant, and others down the field. The play calling has been very conservative, though, under Vic Fangio, and neither Drew Lock nor Teddy Bridgewater feels like anything more than a placeholder for whoever is next.

RED FLAGS

1. **Deshaun Watson, HOU:** Houston brought Tyrod Taylor in this offseason, and it feels like there is a decent chance he will be the starting QB for the Texans to open the season. This organization is at rock bottom, and Deshaun Watson's offseason off-the-field troubles have only made a bad situation worse. When on the field, you know Watson is a top 5 QB talent. "On the field" is the crucial phrase in 2021. The Texans lost J.J. Watt, had very few draft picks, and now have their franchise QB who wants out but is immovable due to scandal. There will be some who see opportunity with Watson at a discount, but there isn't enough information regarding his status to make a fantasy investment right now. If he is acquitted, comes back, and plays with no repercussions, Watson should be between the 6th-8th QB off the board. Otherwise, let someone else roll the dice with their fantasy season.
2. **Taysom Hill/Jameis Winston, NO:** The only worse than running back by committee is quarterback by committee. I find it hard, deep down in my gut, to believe that Sean Payton will roll with Taysom Hill as a full-fledged starting quarterback in the NFL. Jameis Winston has a live arm, and yes, the knock on him is all the interceptions in his Tampa days. In his defense, Bruce Arians' offense is super aggressive, throwing the ball downfield at all times and is prone to high turnover rates. The Saints have Michael Thomas and Alvin Kamara, two of the most efficient weapons in the NFL, who excel after the catch. A dialed-back Jameis Winston could be a better QB than people may realize. The trouble is, there will likely be an increased Taysom Hill workload regardless, and that potentially hurts his fantasy upside, especially in the red zone. The Saints QB situation is a hard pass for me in 2021.

UP AND COMING

1. **Trevor Lawrence, JAC:** Generational talent. There is no "comp" for Trevor Lawrence. He's the best QB prodigy since Peyton Manning, but far more athletic. He has arm strength, speed, awareness. The total package. He's stepping into a team with a fair amount to work with on day one, and he will be the starter in Week 1. Urban Meyer has had success everywhere, but the NFL is a different animal. How the whole thing comes together will be fascinating to watch. However, Trevor Lawrence is worth a top 3 dynasty pick in any format and has the upside to finish as a low-end QB1/high-end QB2 in redraft leagues. The term "can't miss" can be overused, but, it's appropriate when describing Trevor Lawrence.
2. **Trey Lance, SF:** Trey Lance may have sat out last season, but his 2019 college stats and his pro day screamed elite-level talent. I guess that the 49ers will pivot to Lance midway through the '21 season. His sitting out two straight seasons would be detrimental to his development. Lance has Steve McNair-like talent and is a bright student of the game. His film speaks for itself, and I have little concern about his level of competition. He threw 28 TDs with 0 TD's in '19 and rushed for 1,100 yards with 14 rushing TDs in 16 games. He's going to be a fantasy force. Be aggressive in dynasty formats (especially Superflex). In redraft Superflex leagues, he's a draft and stash QB3.
3. **Justin Fields, CHI:** So much for Andy Dalton as QB1! The Bears moved up to draft Justin Fields when he fell in the draft, and he will see the field sooner than later for the Bears. Fields is an accurate passer with a strong arm and speed. He also doesn't shy away from the big stage and is entering a Bears offense with some weapons. The Bears have nowhere to go but up at the quarterback position. You'll hear the Dak Prescott comparisons, but he's quicker than Dak. Fields may even start Week 1 considering what the Bears gave up to get him, but he's more likely fantasy relevant in the latter part of the '21 season.
4. **Zack Wilson, NYJ:** Zack Wilson is flashy and makes some highlight-reel plays. The question remains: how will he fare against better competition than he saw at BYU? And honestly, that's a very fair question. His play-making ability is undeniable, and he's a fiery kid the fans will love. However, it's the higher level of playing quarterback in the NFL that concerns me when it comes to Wilson. We also have no idea what the new Jets offense will look like. I think a wait-and-see approach with Wilson is best for now. He certainly

has upside. I believe talent evaluators have been realistic enough about his downside. He had just as much "unknown" built-in for me as Trey Lance or Justin Fields.

5. **Mac Jones, NE:** If Mac Jones will succeed in the NFL, New England is the most likely spot for him to do so. Jones has a swagger and confidence about him, despite his lack of athleticism (reminiscent of that Tom Brady fellow). Also, like Brady, he doesn't throw on the run well at all. Jones is a pocket passer who needs a clean pocket but has the decision-making skills to be successful. The trouble is, when you look back at his Alabama work, it's easy to look for a 2nd or 3rd option when all of your options are better, faster, more skilled than the opponent's defense. The Pats still lack big-time playmakers. Only time will tell if Jones can elevate the talent around him, or if he has to have elite talent around him to succeed. I think it's 50/50 we see him start the season in '21. I know that sounds a bit aggressive, but this is a first round QB draft pick and Cam Newton didn't dazzle last year with the Pats. Bill Belichick is not going to tolerate losing, especially with Tom brady off winning Super Bowls without him.

6. **Kyle Trask, TB:** He may not have the biggest arm, but Kyle Trask is a big QB that had a lot of success in 2020 for Florida. His footwork needs improvement, and it's unclear if he was a product of the talent around him (like Kyle Pitts and Kadarius Toney) or vice versa. I'm inclined to say the former, not the latter. I also don't expect Trask to see the field the next two seasons. He's a project, not a fantasy investment.

7. **Kellen Mond, MIN:** Like many Texas A&M quarterbacks before him, Kellen Mond can sling the rock. He needs to tighten up the accuracy, sit behind Kirk Cousins for a year, or two, which isn't the worst scenario. He's a work in progress, but he has some upside long-term.

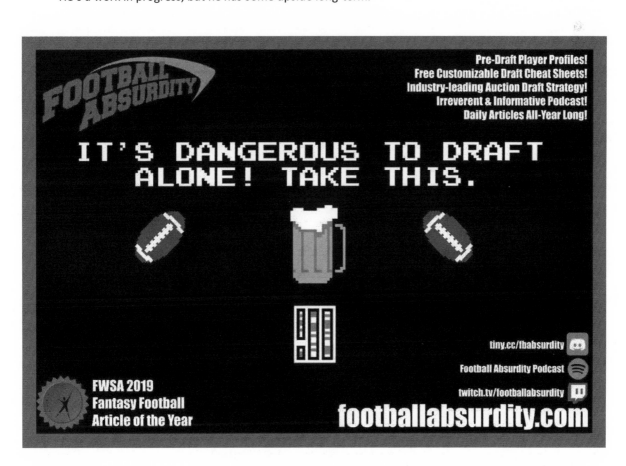

Chapter 5

RUNNING BACKS

Andrew Erickson

PPR SCORING

RB 1 PPR		RPV
1	Christian McCaffrey	42%
2	Dalvin Cook	19%
3	Derrick Henry	15%
4	Alvin Kamara	12%
5	Saquon Barkley	7%
6	Nick Chubb	-9%
7	Ezekiel Elliott	-11%
8	Najee Harris	-13%
9	Aaron Jones	-13%
10	Jonathan Taylor	-16%
11	Austin Ekeler	-16%
12	Joe Mixon	-18%

RB2 PPR		RPV
1	David Montgomery	11%
2	Clyde Edwards-Helaire	8%
3	Antonio Gibson	6%
4	J.K. Dobbins	6%
5	Chris Carson	4%
6	Miles Sanders	4%
7	Darrell Henderson	1%
8	D'Andre Swift	-1%
9	Travis Etienne	-6%
10	Josh Jacobs	-8%
11	Kareem Hunt	-13%
12	Mike Davis	-13%

RB3 PPR		RPV
1	Myles Gaskin	9%
2	Javonte Williams	9%
3	Melvin Gordon	6%
4	Leornard Fournette	3%
5	Ronald Jones	3%
6	Chase Edmonds	3%
7	James Robinson	0%
8	Kenyan Drake	0%
9	David Johnson	-3%
10	Trey Sermon	-6%
11	Damien Harris	-10%
12	Michael Carter	-13%

STANDARD SCORING

RB1 STND		RPV
1	Christian McCaffrey	31%
2	Dalvin Cook	19%
3	Derrick Henry	17%
4	Nick Chubb	4%
5	Aaron Jones	-4%
6	Ezekiel Elliott	-4%
7	Saquon Barkley	-6%
8	Alvin Kamara	-8%
9	Najee Harris	-8%
10	Jonathan Taylor	-10%
11	J.K. Dobbins	-15%
12	David Montgomery	-15%

RB2 STND		RPV
1	Joe Mixon	13%
2	Antonio Gibson	10%
3	Austin Ekeler	10%
4	Chris Carson	7%
5	Clyde Edwards-Helaire	7%
6	Josh Jacobs	-1%
7	D'Andre Swift	-4%
8	Mike Davis	-4%
9	Miles Sanders	-7%
10	Travis Etienne	-9%
11	Myles Gaskin	-9%
12	Darrell Henderson	-12%

RB3 STND		RPV
1	Melvin Gordon	16%
2	Javonte Williams	9%
3	Damien Harris	9%
4	Kareem Hunt	9%
5	David Johnson	2%
6	Ronald Jones	-2%
7	James Robinson	-2%
8	Leornard Fournette	-5%
9	Trey Sermon	-5%
10	James Connor	-9%
11	Chase Edmonds	-9%
12	Kenyan Drake	-13%

*****See Page 3 for information on how to get RPV Cheat Sheets for one-time fee with free updates in July and August after one time purchase***

The rulers of fantasy football have returned: the running backs. Of course, it wasn't so long ago that the fantasy community was selecting the likes of Julio Jones and Antonio Brown over their bell-cow counterparts. Still, a few talented running back draft classes have created a thirst for the position like the golden days.

You'll be hard-pressed to find a league/draft that doesn't feature ten or more RB selected in the first round alone, followed by another eight or nine in the second round. After the first two rounds, drafters enter the dreaded "RB dead-zone," where most appear like workhorses but often have major red flags attached to their profiles. They should be drafted later, but their ADP naturally rises due to the immense scarcity at the position.

Those who don't grab a stud RB will be staring at players like D'Andre Swift, J.K. Dobbins, Miles Sanders, David Montgomery, Josh Jacobs, Myles Gaskin, Mike Davis, or Chase Edmonds as RB1s. Historically speaking, many of the RB drafted in this range fail to pan out — ask those who selected Todd Gurley, James Conner, and Le'Veon Bell in this range last year.

Every fantasy football draft is unique, but one thing's for sure: Running backs are the drivers behind fantasy-winning teams. So, get your studs early, and wait till the later rounds to take shots on running backs in ambiguous backfields. That's where we'll find the next breakout at the position.

THE ELITE

1. **Christian McCaffrey, CAR:** Christian McCaffrey didn't deliver upon his No. 1 overall draft pedigree in 2020, as his season was limited to just three games. The injuries were frustrating for fantasy managers, but at least he was the fantasy superstar we have all come to know and love when he did play. McCaffrey averaged 30.1 fantasy points per game (PPR) and 25.3 touches in his three starts — both ranked first and second at his position. Those numbers weren't too far off from his 2019 stats when he averaged 29.3 fantasy points per game and 25.2 touches per game. Some fantasy managers might be concerned about McCaffrey seeing a lighter load in 2020 to help prevent any future injuries. But everything we saw from the team last year suggests that isn't the case. Instead, the team fed CMC when he was active, and Mike Davis saw an RB1 workload (17.5 touches per game) as a relief runner in Joe Brady's offense. With Davis off to greener pastures in Atlanta, I doubt we see any other Carolina back garner worthwhile looks. Trenton Cannon, Reggie Bonnafon, Rodney Smith, and 2021 fourth-round rookie Chuba Hubbard currently fill out the remainder of the Carolina running back depth chart. CMC was a true difference-maker in 2019, and we should fully expect him to be in the same conversation this season as the Panthers' offense looks to improve in their second year under Brady.

2. **Dalvin Cook, MIN:** Dalvin Cook slots in at No. 2 among the elite after finishing the 2020 season third in fantasy points per game (24.1), second in expected fantasy points per game (21.0), and first in touches per game (25.4). In his fourth season in the league, Cook finished with career-highs in yards per carry (5.0), touchdowns (16), yards after contact per attempt (3.3), and forced missed tackles (72). He finished the year as the league's second-leading rusher with 1,557 rushing yards despite only playing in 14 games. Missing regular-season games has been a consistent trend over Cook's career, as he has yet to play a full 16-game schedule. He played only 14 games in 2019 and 11 in 2018. Injuries aside, Cook's high-end production as a rusher and as a receiver — 40-plus catches the last three seasons — makes up for the fact that he will miss a game or two. His league-leading 26 carries inside the 5-yard line show the offense's heavy reliance on him. The Vikings bolstered their OL this offseason with the additions of Virginia Tech tackle Christian Darrisaw and Ohio State guard Wyatt Davis, so the stage is set for Cook to continue to post elite RB fantasy production. With a workload extremely similar to that of McCaffrey, we shouldn't be surprised to see Cook battle CMC for the No. 1 spot throughout the 2021 season. On paper,

the Vikings' offense looks like a much safer bet to finish as a top-10 unit overall which would vault Cook to become the undisputed RB1 in fantasy football.

3. **Derrick Henry, TEN:** Derrick Henry battered his way into the history books in 2020, rushing for over 2,000 yards and finishing as the league's No. 3 running back in fantasy. In addition, Henry's guaranteed workload is practically unparalleled to other running backs — he saw nearly 25 touches per game in 2020. Volume is the biggest predictor for fantasy success at the running back position, even if the vast majority of touches are carries instead of receptions. So, although we can't project any legitimate pass-game usage for Henry — although the temptation is there based on the Titans' lackluster pass-catching corps— that doesn't hinder him from being a top-five running back. My only concern with him is that he could fall victim to touchdown regression — Henry has scored ten rushing touchdowns over expectation in his last two seasons. And, of course, even a back as great as Henry is unlikely to rip off another 2,000-yard season. Of the seven running backs who have rushed for 2,000 yards, the best fantasy finish the following season was RB5. Five of them finished as top-12 running backs, leaving just two that failed to return RB1 status. The silver lining is that Henry leads all running backs in expected rushing touchdowns (22) over the past two seasons. So even if his touchdown totals regress to the mean, it won't deflate his fantasy value enough to push him out of the top five RBs. You can't go wrong drafting Henry with a top-5 pick, and who knows; maybe new offensive coordinator Todd Downing will target his big back more than the previous regime. In Downing's singular season as an offensive coordinator (2017, Raiders), his offense ranked ninth in targets to running backs.

4. **Saquon Barkley, NYG:** Like CMC, Saquon Barkley's 2020 season was cut short by injuries. He only played in one full game — and it was an utter disaster. Barkley rushed for just six measly yards on 15 carries against the Steelers. Yuck. The Week 1 matchup was brutal, but things started to look up in Week 2 versus the Chicago Bears. Barkley ripped off a long 18-yard gain and appeared on his way to validating the No. 2 overall pick in fantasy drafts. Alas, he went down with a season-ending injury soon after. Entering the 2021 season, Barkley should be all systems go based on his lengthy recovery time, so fantasy managers should not be overly concerned with health. The Giants don't seem overly concerned as they recently exercised the fifth-year option on the running back. In eight games with Daniel Jones in 2019, Barkley averaged 19.5 fantasy points per game — seventh-best at the position. The state of the New York Giants' offense led by vanilla offensive coordinator Jason Garrett is a potential worry, but the situation is not as dire as people make it out to be. Recall that backup Wayne Gallman ranked as the RB10 from Weeks 7-13 last season, averaging 15.8 fantasy points per game. If a backup running back could put up top-10 numbers in last year's Giants' offense, Barkley can easily reclaim his status as a top-three fantasy football RB. The offensive line could also easily improve with starting linemen Andrew Thomas and Matt Peart entering Year 2.

TOP TALENT

1. **Alvin Kamara, NO:** There's a strong argument to be made that Alvin Kamara should be in the elite tier. After all, he finished the 2020 season second in points per game (24.2) and third in expected fantasy points per game (20.5). From a total fantasy points perspective, he finished as the undisputed No. 1 running back. Kamara hauled in a career-high 83 passes, continuing his streak of at least 81 receptions in four straight seasons. Of course, posting elite receiving numbers is nothing new for Kamara. Still, we have to exclude him from the top tier because of the uncertainty of the New Orleans Saints' quarterback situation. We all saw the insane drop-off in receiving numbers with Taysom Hill under center. Kamara's fantasy points per game fell from 27.4 with Drew Brees to 14.2 with Hill. I don't anticipate Hill being the starter come Week 1, but any other quarterback who isn't noodle-armed Brees is bound to impact Kamara's receiving totals negatively. Most signs suggest that Jameis Winston is the frontrunner to take over, and his ability to throw downfield (No.1 aDOT since 2019) could hurt Kamara's bottom line as a receiver. That regression wouldn't be shocking, as Kamara led the NFL in fantasy points scored above

expectation in 2020. He could be forced to make up more production as a rusher. Sean Payton leaned more on his star running back on the ground at the end of the 2020 season. Kamara set a career-high in rushing attempts in Week 16 (22) and then did one better during the wildcard playoff game (23).

2. **Nick Chubb, CLE** Nick Chubb is one of the best pure running backs in the NFL. He finished the regular season first in yards after contact per attempt (4.0) and second in rushing attempts of 15-plus yards (15) despite only being healthy for 11 games. He was so efficient creating yards after contact that his OL ranked 28th in yards before contact — a stat indicating poor offensive line play. But, considering PFF graded the Browns as the No. 1 blocking unit last season, it's much more telling of how talented Chubb truly is. In the full games he played in 2020, Chubb averaged 18.7 fantasy points per game — seventh-best at the position. He was able to accomplish such a feat while averaging just 17 touches per game. Teammate Kareem Hunt played a prominent role in Chubb's low touch volume, as he averaged just under 15 touches per game. It's a credit to Chubb's immense talent that he can produce high-end numbers without the same type of workload other RB1s see. He never played more than 62% of his team's offensive snaps. The Browns' running back would easily have the ceiling of the overall RB1 if anything were to happen to Hunt. His consistency since entering the NFL — three seasons averaging over 5.0 yards per carry and top-four PFF grade — is truly remarkable. Drafting Chubb at the backend of the first round/top of the second round is highway robbery for a player of his caliber. Especially considering the Browns have the easiest strength of schedule for running backs in 2021. With back-to-back layups to open the year (Chiefs, Texans), expect Chubb to start out of the gates "en Fuego."

3. **Aaron Jones, GB:** Aaron Jones has been nothing short of fantastic since entering the NFL in 2017, ranking third in PFF rushing grade (91.1) and fourth in yards per carry (5.1). Last year Jones was stellar; he rushed for a career-high 1,230 yards (5.6 yards per attempt) and ranked fourth in the league in yards after contact per attempt (3.6). It's hard not to view Jones as a top-10 fantasy RB considering how efficient he has been. After finishing the 2019 season as the RB2 overall, Jones came in as the RB5 in 2020 while working in a timeshare. He finished this past season 12th in touches per game (17.7). At age 26 and with 846 touches on his resume, Jones has at least a couple more super-productive fantasy seasons within him. And playing in one of the league's most high-powered offenses led by Aaron Rodgers raises the floor. Not to mention that Jones' "thorn in his side" in the form of Jamaal Williams is no longer with the team. Williams' departure can only ooze optimism for Jones' continued work as one of the team's most reliable receivers. The Packers' running back has at least 47 receptions in back-to-back seasons with Williams in the fold. There's no guarantee that A.J. Dillon immediately steps into that role and demands a significant target share.

4. **Joe Mixon, CIN:** Joe Mixon was a usage monster through the first six weeks of the season. He ranked second in the league in carries (20 per game), ninth in routes run (21 per game), and 15th in targets (four per game). His overall touches per game (23.3) during the regular season ranked fourth-highest among all running backs. The heavy workload helped him finish 11th in fantasy points per game (16.9) and fifth in expected fantasy points per game (18.1). Mixon's poor yards per carry (3.6) figure and lack of explosive runs — only three runs of 15-plus yards — tarnished his efficiency metrics in 2020, but the 25-year-old is far from washed up. Breakaway run rate is highly volatile, and there's no doubt that Mixon would have broken off more big runs if he suited up for more games. In 2018 and 2019, Mixon ranked second and fourth, respectively, in rushes of 15-plus yards. The former second-rounder has bounce-back written all over him for 2021 as quarterback Joe Burrow heads into Year 2. Cincinnati's offensive line is improved, and the days of Giovani stealing targets are long gone. With a horrible defense returning, the Bengals are shaping up to be this year's version of the 2020 Dallas Cowboys — shootouts and offensive fireworks as far as the eye can see. If that ends up being the case, Mixon will have his hands full in fantasy points and more than pay off his early second-round ADP. The only problem with Mixon is the timetable on Burrow's recovery from the ACL injury. Combine that uncertainty with three brutal matchups to start the year (Vikings, Bears, Steelers), and we could see Mixon start slow...again. Luckily the matchups change for the better Weeks 4-6 with the Jaguars, Packers, and Lions.

5. **Ezekiel Elliott, DAL:** Ezekiel Elliott's 2020 season is one he would like to forget. After starting the year red hot with Dak Prescott under center (22.6 fantasy points per game, third), his numbers plummeted (12.9 fantasy points per game, 26th). Losing Dak was significant for Zeke's fantasy stock, but we can't forget the rotating carousel that was the Dallas Cowboys offensive line, which sustained multiple injuries throughout the season. As a result, they finished the year as PFF's fourth-lowest-graded run-blocking team (57.2). The cards were utterly stacked against Elliott in 2020. He finished with the most fantasy points under expectation (-49.8) at the running back position, but those numbers tend to regress positively. Presumably, with Prescott and a healthier offensive line returning in 2021, we should see Zeke return to the upper echelon of fantasy running backs. So the high-end usage is probably still going to be there despite what Tony Pollard truthers might say. Let's not forget that Elliott led the NFL in carries inside the 5-yard line (26) but only converted five into scores. In 2019, he had 18 carries inside the 5-yard line and scored ten touchdowns. Everything about Elliott's 2020 campaign screams that he's about to run head-first into a bounce-back 2021 season.

6. **Austin Ekeler, LAC:** Like many top-tier running backs in 2020, Austin Ekeler was plagued by injuries. He missed a huge chunk of the season (Weeks 4-11), and that has soured many on his potential in 2021. But we can't forget that he was the RB7 before his injury (Weeks 1-3) and the RB7 upon returning from his injury (Weeks 12-16). In eight games played with Justin Herbert under center, Ekeler averaged 19.1 fantasy points (sixth) and 18.3 touches per game (ninth). His per-game pace with Herbert would have put him over 100 catches in a 16-game season. Ekeler is still the same back that fantasy managers rejoiced over in 2019 when he finished as the RB4 overall. The only difference now is that he has an entirely revamped offensive line from a season ago. That year's unit was PFF's 32nd-ranked run-blocking group. The additions of center Corey Linsley, guard Matt Feiler and first-round rookie tackle Rashawn Slater are massive upgrades. With only the likes of second-year runner Joshua Kelley, veteran Justin Jackson and rookie plodder Larry Rountree competing for touches in the Chargers' backfield, it's safe to say that Ekeler is looking forward to a healthy workload in 2021.

SOLID OPTIONS

1. **David Montgomery, CHI:** David Montgomery finished the year with 301 touches (20 per game), which ranked fourth among all running backs. Tarik Cohen's injury certainly helped vault Montgomery to RB1 status, especially down the stretch — he was RB1 overall from Week 12 on — but Monty would have likely flirted with 250 total touches either way. We simply can't ignore young RBs with guaranteed volume, even if they aren't exciting names or are athletic freaks. This is especially true when they're being drafted at their floors. And although Montgomery is often the punch-line for "unathletic RBs," his elusiveness is vastly underrated. I believed his broken tackle ability would eventually translate into more big runs, and that's exactly what transpired last season. As a result, he racked up over 100 more rushing yards on carries of 15-plus yards compared to 2019. Heading into the 2020 season, Montgomery's ADP was hovering around RB23. He was a value then, and he's currently being drafted in a similar range meaning his price is already factoring in the return of Cohen.

2. **Chris Carson, SEA:** Chris Carson's current ADP is absolutely egregious. Returning as the clear-cut workhorse for the Seattle Seahawks in 2021, he has easy RB1 fantasy potential. We know that the Seahawks have an affinity for establishing the run, and Carson has been the clear bell cow whenever he has been healthy. Carson was a top-eight fantasy running back through the first six weeks of the 2020 season, averaging 20 fantasy points per game (seventh) and 16.5 expected fantasy points per game (13th) while playing a 56% snap share. His injury history is well-documented, but his production when healthy is too good to pass on.

3. **Myles Gaskin, MIA:** The Miami Dolphins predictably did not draft a running back until the seventh round (Gerrid Doaks), which is a huge win for Myles Gaskin. He appears locked-and-loaded to resume the RB1 status he earned last season when healthy. The Miami coaching staff seems to love Gaskin — his 18.3

touches per game ranked ninth at the running back position. The Dolphins' second-year runner missed time after contracting COVID-19 but slid right back into a starting role upon returning in Week 16, commanding a 75% snap share and 19 total touches. He finished sixth in expected fantasy points per game (17.6) and 12th in fantasy points per game (16.8) from Weeks 1-17. His impressive per-game rates were buoyed by his second-ranked average yards per route run (1.87), which trailed only Alvin Kamara (2.19) during the regular season. The Dolphins look to be an offense rising in 2021, and the 24-year-old Gaskin figures to be a major beneficiary.

4. **Mike Davis, ATL:** The Atlanta Falcons failed to draft a running back, signing only UDFA Javian Hawkins. Big Mike looks poised to be a solid fantasy contributor for a second straight year. In 12 games as the Panthers' full-blown starter in 2020, Davis averaged 15.4 fantasy points (15th), 16.7 expected fantasy points (10th), and 17.4 touches per game (14th). He does not generate explosive plays, but he's a capable pass-catcher and should see plenty of goal-line touches in a high-powered offense. Todd Gurley's exit from the Atlanta Falcons' offense leaves nearly three-quarters of the team's goal-line touches up for grabs in 2021. Recall that Gurley was the RB6 through the first nine weeks of the season, averaging a rushing touchdown per game in Atlanta's high-powered offense. With Davis entrenched as the lead back, it's hard to envision him not stumbling into fantasy production. Just be wary that it might not happen right away. Three of his first five matchups to start the season are against defenses that ranked top-10 versus RBs in fantasy points allowed.

5. **Kareem Hunt, CLE:** Kareem Hunt finished the 2020 season as the RB10 overall and the RB23 in fantasy points per game (13.7). The Cleveland Brown's 1B running back totaled over 1,100 yards from scrimmage (1,145) and filled in admirably when Nick Chubb went down in Week 4. Hunt operated as the team's workhorse averaging 17.2 touches, 14.7 fantasy points, and 13.8 expected fantasy points per game for the five weeks of games that followed. As the clear-cut leader of the backfield, Hunt got a slight boost from a larger workload, but make no mistake. He was still a great fantasy producer, even when working in tandem with Chubb. In the 13 games (including postseason) the Browns' duo played together, Hunt averaged 12.8 touches, 13.4 fantasy points, and 12.2 expected fantasy points per game. A 60-40 split in Chubb's favor will undoubtedly hinder Hunt's RB1 potential, but you'll be hard-pressed to find another RB2 in an NFL backfield involved as much as he is. Hunt also seems to be the slight favorite as the team's preferred option on passing downs. He out-targeted Chubb (40 vs. 28) in games they played together. Additionally, Hunt garnered the vast majority of snaps on third down (84%).

RED FLAGS

1. **J.K. Dobbins, BAL:** J.K. Dobbins was spectacular down the stretch as a rookie, finishing as RB11 from Weeks 11-17 in full PPR. But, running backs tied to a mobile quarterback are often short-changed when it comes to the passing game. As well as Dobbins performed for fantasy from Weeks 11-17, J.D. McKissic came in one spot ahead of him because he caught 37 passes. Dobbins caught three. Dobbins' outlook would look better if he were the clear-cut workhorse, but that's not likely the case with Gus Edwards in the mix. Edwards didn't see fewer than seven carries in a game after Week 13. He also was only slightly out-touched by Dobbins (74 to 86) during that time. Not to mention, Dobbins ran extremely hot when it came to scoring touchdowns. He scored at least one touchdown in every game from Week 11 onward. Unfortunately, that's not likely going to be sustainable.

2. **Josh Jacobs, LV:** Josh Jacobs was by far the biggest-name running back to take a huge value hit during free agency. The Las Vegas Raiders signed Kenyan Drake, and that means Jacobs' path to becoming an RB1 seems extremely unlikely. Drake's hefty contract guarantees he will see the field more than any other running back Jacobs has shared a backfield with in the past. Drake's pass-catching chops also ensure that Jacobs' receiving usage won't be something fantasy gamers can rely on week-to-week. Not including, the Raiders completely overhauled their starting offensive line. They moved on from three of last season's starters — Gabe Jackson, Rodney Hudson, Trent Brown — to save space against the salary

cap. In addition, they added tackle Alex Leatherwood in the draft, but it remains to be seen how the new offensive line will gel in their first year together. We can't view Jacobs as anything more than a low-end RB2 heading into 2021, especially with the Las Vegas Raiders facing the most challenging schedule based on Vegas implied win totals. Additionally, negative game scripts are not favorable for Jacobs because he doesn't project much volume in the passing game. He needs touchdowns, and those might be in short supply. Thirty-one percent of Jacobs' fantasy points last season came from touchdowns, the 10th-highest mark in the league.

3. **Miles Sanders, PHI:** Miles Sanders will be the first Philadelphia player drafted in fantasy football next season, but I have even more concerns about him with Hurts under center. I've done extensive research on mobile quarterback influence on running back production — the reality is that it's going to be tough for Sanders to finish as a top-12 fantasy RB without a heavy receiving workload. And mobile QBs like Hurts don't have to dump the ball off to RBs when they can scramble just as quickly. Perhaps it's still possible that Sanders could make up the difference as a pure rusher on the ground, as the mobile QB "opens lanes of RBs" corollary has proven true in the last two seasons. But the increased efficiency on rushing attempts doesn't always make up for the lack of volume for running backs, which we know reigns supreme at the position. So Sanders will have to continue his upward trajectory of efficiency and ramp up his rushing production to become a worthwhile pick in the third round. The Eagles also drafted Kenneth Gainwell in the fifth round, and he should dramatically affect Sanders' role in the passing game. Gainwell has already been dubbed the team's "Nyheim Hines," per head coach Nick Sirianni. Hines finished third in receptions at the running back position last season (64).

4. **Chase Edmonds, ARZ:** The Arizona Cardinals were another team rumored to be in the market for a running back but passed. Instead, the backfield belongs to Chase Edmonds and James Conner, with Edmonds the favorite to be the more featured player. Still, it's important to call out that the addition of dynamic slot receiver Rondale Moore may dampen expectations on the receiving volume for any Cardinals running back. Moore's YAC-ability should draw targets close to the line of scrimmage, an overlap that will likely limit RB receiving production in Kliff Kingsbury's horizontal Air Raid offense. No RB saw a higher percentage of snaps from the slot than Edmonds did in 2020 (26%). Let's also not forget that Kyler Murray's mobility already makes RB targets scarce. The other concern for Edmonds is his lack of potential goal-line work. Seventy percent of Arizona's carries inside the 5-yard line are available, which presents a golden opportunity for whoever can claim the role. But if history tells us anything, it won't be Edmonds. Over the past two seasons, Edmonds has only one goal-line carry. Since 2018, Conner has 32. Last season, Kenyan Drake's fantasy value was heavily connected to his work at the goal line — his 21 rushing attempts inside the 5-yard line tied for the third-most in the league — but those touches might not even exist in the 2021 Cardinals' offense. Drake's increased role near the goal line directly correlated with an injury Murray suffered around Week 7. From Weeks 11-16, Drake totaled nearly 72% of his goal-line attempts (15), while Murray had just two carries. During the first ten weeks of the season, Murray and Drake were tied with six rushing attempts inside the 5-yard line. Assuming Murray stays healthy in 2021, Edmonds looks to be third on the totem pole to get any work at the goal line. Like Jacobs, 31% of Drake's fantasy production also came from touchdowns.

5. **Raheem Mostert, SF:** Raheem Mostert looked to be in a prime spot to be a sneaky RB1 candidate in 2021, but things didn't quite play out in his favor. Not only did the 49ers draft Trey Sermon in the third round, but they also selected Elijah Mitchell a few rounds later. I fully expect Mostert to be the Day 1 starter, but his chances of hanging onto the role all year are dwindling with the team's investment in Sermon. Last season, Mostert averaged 15 touches per game (22nd), which was more than any other 49ers RB. Wilson averaged 12.6 touches, with Jerick McKinnon (7.6), Tevin Coleman (4.0), and JaMycal Hasty (6.6) trailing behind. Since the start of 2019, Mostert ranks second in yards per attempt (5.5), sixth in yards after contact per attempt (3.3), and sixth in rushing attempts of 15-plus yards (24). Mostert's a fine running back to acquire at a cheap price, but like many other older running backs, his shelf life as a

long-term fantasy producer isn't for the faint of heart. Mostert will need to stay healthy and maintain uber-productivity to fend off the other 49ers' running backs vying for touches.

6. **Melvin Gordon III, DEN:** Melvin Gordon III never saw a 60-plus percent snap share last season in games when Phillip Lindsay was healthy (not including games with Kendall Hinton at QB). That suggests Gordon and Javonte Williams will operate in some kind of 60-40 snap split, which should be more than enough for Williams to prove he is the more worthy RB1. After all, Williams spent nearly his entire collegiate career playing in a committee, so he's more than up for the challenge. MG3 is an expiring RB asset, and with no ties to the new general manager George Paton, you're much better off letting somebody else draft him. His 13.8 fantasy points per game didn't even crack top-20 running back fantasy production.

7. **James Robinson, JAX:** The addition of Travis Etienne drastically hit James Robinson's stock, and anybody holding out hope that J-Rob is still going to retain any kind of consistent fantasy value will be highly disappointed next season. The new coaching staff has no attachments to him, and the volume he received last season that vaulted him to RB1 status is nothing more than a distant memory.The real driver behind Robinson's fantasy success — like most running backs — was sheer volume in 2020. His 96% of team RB carries in the 14 games he played was the most in the league last season. In his historic 2019 season, Christian McCaffrey's mark was 93%. Robinson's final team running back opportunity share — combining RB carries and targets — was 73%, which ranked second to Derrick Henry. The 2020 Jacksonville Jaguars fed Robinson more than any other running back in the NFL. So it's hard to blame when the team's depth chart was rounded out by Ryquell Armstead, Chris Thompson, Dare Ogunbowale, and Devine Ozigbo. With the running back room revamped in 2021, Robinson's chances at returning to reliable fantasy value will be extremely low. Not to mention that Carlos Hyde has also been thrown into the Jaguars' RB rotation, and he shouldn't be overlooked. Wherever Hyde has played the past few seasons — Seattle, Houston, Cleveland, Jacksonville — he has found a way to garner touches and opportunities. And let's not forget that Jacksonville offensive coordinator Darrell Bevell was the play-caller for the Detroit Lions last season. The same offense operated a committee involving Adrian Peterson, Kerryon Johnson, and D'Andre Swift despite the rookie outplaying the others. There are many different ways that this backfield shakes out next year, but the writings on the wall that Robinson might be the one left holding the bag wondering where everything went wrong.

8. **Damien Harris, NE:** The Patriots selected Rhamondre Stevenson in the fourth round, and he joins a backfield that fantasy gamers have come to know too well, as one that can be pretty frustrating to decipher. Adding the massive back is a tell-tale sign that Sony Michel's days are numbered in New England — the team also declined Michel's fifth-year option. Either way, Damien Harris has to be hands-off in drafts despite his success running the football last season. There's no telling how this backfield will shake out, and Harris doesn't have a ton of fantasy upside with Cam Newton vulturing touchdowns. Despite being one of the lone bright spots for the Patriots in 2021, he only averaged 9.1 fantasy points per game (41st) because he had only five catches and scored just two rushing touchdowns. In addition, Cam Newton's rushing ability inside the 5-yard line put a massive damper on Harris' fantasy upside. As we project into 2021, all the issues that were holding back Harris are still in the fold. He doesn't have the chance to see an uptick in pass-game work with James White, and there's heavy competition for goal-line duties. I'd much rather take a shot on Stevenson several rounds later and hope that Belichick uses him as a boomer version of LeGarrette Blount. The Oklahoma senior ranks second since 2019 in yards after contact per attempt (4.7) among 2021 draft-eligible running backs.

9. **David Johnson, HOU:** As the presumed starter for the Houston Texans, on the surface, David Johnson looks like a great value in the mid-to-late rounds of fantasy drafts. But there's a reason why he is going so late. The Texans' offense has disaster written all over them in 2021. Houston has major question marks at quarterback. So, they brought in Tyrod Taylor and drafted Davis Mills as their contingency plan, with Deshaun Watson's situation unresolved. To make matters worse, the team also signed former Denver Broncos running back Phillip Lindsay. So, we could be looking at the league's ugliest three-headed monster in 2021 between Johnson, Mark Ingram II, and Lindsay. Throw in that he is already 29 years old,

coming off a season in which he posted an unsustainable breakaway run rate, and I can't help but think he's the next coming of Todd Gurley II, Mark Ingram, Matt Breida, Tevin Coleman, and Le'Veon Bell.

10. **Leonard Fournette, TB:** 2020 was a second to forget for Leonard Fournette — at least it was till he completed his Super Saiyan transformation into "Playoff Lenny" down the stretch for the Tampa Bay Buccaneers. The one formerly known as "Fat Lenny" averaged 21.7 fantasy points, 20.5 touches, and 5.3 targets per game from the Wild Card Round to Super Bowl Sunday. Although, his overly impressive playoff performance overshadows the fact that he was horrible during the regular season. He averaged 12.2 fantasy points per game (29th) and was inferior to Ronald Jones as a rusher. Fournette averaged 3.8 yards per attempt (45th), while Jones averaged 5.1 yards per attempt despite running behind the same offensive line. The veteran back saw most of his fantasy points stem from receiving production — 54 receptions, 67 targets — but his locked-and-loaded pass-catching role is in question with the team's addition of Giovani Bernard. Joe Mixon-truthers are too familiar with Gio because he tends to limit starting RB fantasy production due to his receiver and pass-blocker skills. Per PFF, Bernard finished last season as the third-highest graded pass-blocker. Fournette finished 41st out of 42 qualifying running backs. LF's chances to lead this backfield in touches don't look as clear-cut as the consensus believes.

11. **Jeff Wilson Jr, SF:** *Wilson will miss open to the season with a torn meniscus in his knee. Tevin Coleman and Jerick McKinnon are no longer with the 49ers, leaving the backfield to Raheem Mostert, Jeff Wilson Jr., Wayne Gallman, JaMycal Hasty, and rookies Trey Sermon and Elijah Mitchell. Talk about a crowded backfield. Mostert (12.7 points per game) and Wilson (13.3 points per game) posted almost identical fantasy production when given the opportunity in 2020. But, Mostert will be drafted first across fantasy circles under the assumption that he'll be the starter, with Sermon likely hot on his tail as the incoming hot-shot rookie. Fantasy gamers proclaiming to know for sure who will start in arguably the most volatile backfield in all of fantasy football are making a bet with some long odds attached. During Weeks 16 and 17, Wilson played snap shares of 68% and 83%, with Mostert sidelined. Mostert never played a snap share higher than 59% during the regular season. Wilson also rushed for 259 yards in that final two-game stretch and caught four of eight targets for 33 yards with two scores. There's a non-zero chance that Wilson ends up being the starter for a solid stretch of games at some point during the season. Injuries happen — especially to 49ers running backs — and Wilson has a nose for production whenever he is thrust into an expanded role. He scored ten touchdowns despite only playing three games with a 50-plus percent snap share. In those contests, he averaged 27.7 fantasy points per game. When Wilson/Mostert were healthy for four weeks toward the end of the season, Wilson out-carried Mostert at the goal line (six versus four) and out-snapped him in the red zone. In such a crowded backfield, Wilson is sure to get overlooked. Last year, he finished eighth (tied with Aaron Jones) in fantasy points per snap (0.47).

UP AND COMING

1. **Johnathan Taylor, IND:** Jonathan Taylor cemented himself as a first-round pick in 2021 fantasy drafts by the time the 2020 regular season ended, but it was a rollercoaster ride for him to reach this point. He started with a bang, rushing for 57 yards or more in his first five starts after Marlon Mack went down with an injury. The rookie then flamed out after the team's Week 7 bye, outplayed by backup Jordan Wilkins for several weeks.The team didn't give up on Taylor despite the downturn, and he got back on track versus the Green Bay Packers in Week 11. From that point to Week 17, Taylor was the RB3 overall and averaged 26.1 fantasy points per game — tops at the position over that stretch. Finishing as the overall RB1 is well within Taylor's range of outcomes with his talented skillset. The only question surrounds Taylor's role and how he might operate as a pass-catcher in conjunction with Nyheim Hines. I wouldn't necessarily give Taylor a massive boost as receiver heading into 2021 with a much more mobile Carson Wentz under center in place of the statuesque Philip Rivers. Mobile quarterbacks tend to target their RBs in the pass-game less frequently, so temper expectations regarding Taylor's ability to outperform his receiving production from a season ago unless he completely supplants Hines in the

passing game. During Taylor's final seven games, he ran one more route than Hines (105 vs. 104) but saw eight fewer targets (20 vs. 28). But even in a timeshare, Taylor should still see plenty of volume. Throughout his tumultuous rookie season, he finished eighth in total touches (268) and 11th in touches per game (17.7). That usage was more than enough to land him ninth in fantasy points per game (16.9), sixth in PFF grade, and third in the NFL in rushing yards (1,169).

2. **Najee Harris, PIT:** Let me introduce rookie running back Najee Harris — the Pittsburgh Steelers' next three-down bell cow for those who aren't familiar with him. With similar size and pass-catching ability to Le'Veon Bell, Pittsburgh selected a do-it-all running back in the first round of this year's draft. During his senior season, Harris racked up 1,464 rushing yards and 26 touchdowns on 252 carries. His 43 receptions on 53 targets were career highs, and he ranked third in the nation at the running back position. He dropped only one target and forced a league-high 22 missed tackles after the catch. The primary concern for Harris and the Pittsburgh offense is the team's offensive line, but that's been blown out of proportion when it comes to the stud RB. Volume trumps efficiency at the running back position in fantasy football. Since 2012, the correlation coefficient between RB fantasy points scored and touches (0.72) drastically outweighs the same metric between RB fantasy points scored and PFF run-blocking grade (0.26). The Alabama product will be fed with touches in the Steelers offense, putting him firmly in high-end RB2 fantasy territory. He's easily a top-15 fantasy RB in 2021. Last year, we saw James Conner average top-15 fantasy numbers whenever he saw at least 12 touches. With the return of tackle Zach Banner (lost to an ACL injury in 2020) and the addition of rookie center Kendrick Green (replacement for Maurkice Pouncey), the Steel Curtain OL can also be much-improved from a season ago. Harris' opening schedule is also highly favorable. His first four matchups to start the year: Buffalo Bills, Las Vegas Raiders, Cincinnati Bengals, and Green Bay Packers. Fade him at your own risk.

3. **Antonio Gibson, WAS:** Antonio Gibson entered the NFL with just 33 collegiate careers on his resume, which goes to show how impressive he was in 2021. The WFT rookie running back finished as the RB14 overall and averaged 14.7 fantasy points per game (19th) on the back 11 rushing touchdowns (sixth-most). He also finished as PFF's fifth-highest graded rusher (85.3) primarily because of his fifth-ranked missed tackle rate (22%) and No. 1 ranked stuff rate (4.1%). In addition, no running back had a smaller percentage of his rushing attempts for no gain or a loss than Gibson. There's plenty to like about Gibson's fantasy prospects heading into 2021 with an expanded role in his range of outcomes. He only reached or surpassed a 44 percent snap share in eight games last season. In those contests, AG averaged 17.7 fantasy points per game (seventh) and 17.2 touches per game (14th). If The Football Team opts to involve Gibson more looks in the passing game — an area he should thrive in considering he played WR in college — he's got a chance to be the No. 1 fantasy running back from the 2020 draft class. We got a glimpse of Gibson's true potential back in Week 12 versus Dallas —Twenty carries, seven targets, and over 36 fantasy points. With Washington's offense on an upward trajectory led by Ryan Fitzpatrick under center, Gibson's got megastar potential written all over him.

4. **D'Andre Swift, DET:** The Detroit Lions added running back depth in free agency by inking Jamaal Williams to a two-year deal. The initial reaction from the fantasy football community seems to be that this is a hit to D'Andre Swift's fantasy draft stock, but I'm not sure I agree. Only a select few elite running backs don't split snaps with a teammate to some extent. So projecting Swift to see a 60% snap share with Williams is hardly a strong reason to fade him. Williams hovered around a 30% to 50% snap share with Green Bay last year, and that didn't stop Aaron Jones from becoming a locked-and-loaded RB1 every week. Sure, it would have been nice for Jones to have seen a 90% snap share, but then his body might have broken down, or he might have been less efficient. Swift finished his rookie season 18th in RB points per game (14.9) despite seeing a 70-plus percent snap share only once. Even with Williams in the fold, Swift will probably be the clear touch and snap leader in the Lions' backfield, making him worth buying at an ADP discount. New HC Dan Campbell and offensive coordinator Anthony Lynn come from offenses where their true RB1 wasn't an every-snap player. Instead, running backs Alvin Kamara and Austin Ekeler saw snap shares between 50% and 70% in 2020, which is the exact type of workload we can project for Swift

in 2021.Those concerned that Williams will eat into Swift's pass-game usage shouldn't be. Adrian Peterson (12) and Kerryon Johnson (19) combined for the same number of receptions as Williams (31) last season. Swift doesn't necessarily benefit from the Williams signing (we want all the touches). Still, savvy fantasy gamers can take advantage of a potential discount on a second-year player with superstar potential. The larger concern for his outlook is the potential lack of touchdowns. I'm not particularly excited about the Detroit Lions' offense with Jared Goff under center. But there's a possibility that Goff's presence ends up making Swift a value in PPR formats come draft season. Non-mobile quarterbacks tend to target running backs more in the passing game than QBs who rush the ball — that's becoming an important factor when so many of the game's best QBs offer at least some rushing skill. Last season, Swift was 12th in targets (56) and seventh in yards per route run (1.58) among RBs. He barely trailed Austin Ekeler in both categories. Ekeler always saw heavy usage in the passing game during the Lynn era in San Diego/Los Angeles. Swift's high-end pass-game usage could easily vault the talented second-year back to low-end RB1 status by the end of 2021.

5. **Clyde Edwards-Helaire, KC:** I can't envision any scenario where the Chiefs bring back Le'Veon Bell after he was a complete afterthought in their offense and essentially benched in favor of Darrel Williams. It wasn't until Bell arrived in Kansas City that we started to see Clyde Edwards-Helaire's fantasy production falter. During the first six weeks of the season, CEH was the RB11 overall, averaging 15.9 fantasy points per game (17th), 18.3 expected fantasy points per game (seventh), and an absurd 21.3 touches per game. His 505 rushing yards over the start of the season ranked second in the league. With only Williams and Jerick McKinnon as "threats" for touches in the backfield, Edwards-Helaire is the exact post-hype running back to target in 2021. He failed to meet the impossible expectations placed on him a year ago as a first-round pick, which is why he's now readily available in the third round. The Kansas City offensive line went from broke to rich in just a few short months, which can only bode well for CEH's fantasy upside in 2021. All the reasons we liked him last season are still firmly in place; he's just finally priced appropriately.

6. **Travis Etienne, JAX:** Rookie Travis Etienne should be viewed as the clear favorite to lead the team in RB snaps — first-round RBs don't sit. The backfield will start as a committee, but Etienne will benefit the most from receptions and goal-line work. That usage puts the rookie into low-end RB2 territory, whereas James Robinson's ranking plummets from solid RB2 to outside the top-30. Etienne's experience as a goal-line back (most carries inside the 5-yard line since 2018) combined with his receiving prowess (12% target share last season) ensures that even just 12-15 touches per game will be of the fantasy-friendly variety. We cannot get too wrapped up in the Robinson/Carlos Hyde RB debacle but should zoom out enough to see the bigger picture. Etienne is attached to his college QB Trevor Lawrence, who he connected with for over 100 receptions at Clemson. That's a *great* situation for him to be in. As Urban Meyer said, Etienne is going to be the third-down back. So he will be involved heavily in the passing game, and we cherish that in PPR formats.Temper expectations with ETN to start the year, with the mindset that you'll likely have a fringe RB1 by the time the fantasy playoffs come knocking.

7. **Darrell Henderson/*Cam Akers OUT FOR THE SEASON WITH ACHILLIES TEAR*** The Rams' rookie running back did everything in his power to position himself as a top-10 running back in 2021. He posted solid rushing statistics despite facing the second-most stacked fronts (52%) and consistently earned 18-plus opportunities once he finally became the team's true workhorse in Week 13. During that stretch, Akers averaged 16.6 fantasy points per game and 18.4 expected fantasy points per game. He underperformed versus expectation because he fell short in the touchdown department. He only scored three rushing touchdowns, in part because he posted a goose egg (0-for-6) inside the 5-yard line. Jared Goff scored more rushing touchdowns (two) inside the 5-yard line. Matthew Stafford's arrival in L.A. was icing on the cake for Akers' upside, that was until he tore his Achilles in July. Now, Darrell Henderson will get a crack at the starting job and is line for a ton of volume. Henderson excelled at times last year and his speed is not a problem. However, it's still unclear what other names could be brought into camp to compete for carries in 2021.

8. **Javonte Williams, DEN:** The ultimate tackle-breaking running back has found a new home in Denver. Javonte Williams' missed tackle rate per attempt (48%) was 12 percentage points higher than the next running back in 2020. The superior missed tackle rate is eerily similar to that of Washington Football Team running back Antonio Gibson during his final season at Memphis. The only difference is that Gibson totaled just 71 touches compared to Williams' 181. Gibson was arguably one of the most efficient RBs in the league last year, finishing second in fantasy points per snap among all RBs. Williams graded as PFF's No. 1 inside zone/power runner (92.3) last season, and that makes him a perfect fit for Denver's offense. The Broncos finished second in inside zone/power runs in 2020. With Denver spending a high Day 2 pick (and trading up) to add Williams, we should expect him to finally see the type of workload that will unleash his vast talent as a true all-purpose back. MG3 is entering the final year of his contract, so his days appear to be numbered in the Mile High City. We saw the Broncos divvy snaps between MG3 and Phillip Lindsay at 60-40 clip, so starting with that split seems like a realistic projection. But, Williams' explosiveness — second in the nation in runs of 15-plus yards — is going to help him usurp Gordon as the team's lead back sooner rather than later. As a result, he should be viewed as a low-end RB2 — ahead of the veteran — heading into 2021.

9. **Trey Sermon, SF:** Trey Sermon's draft capital has vaulted him to the clear-cut RB4 among the rookie class, giving him a decent chance of becoming a fantasy factor in the 49ers' offense. Sermon averaged 7.7 yards per carry and earned the fourth-best PFF rushing grade (88.9) on outside-zone concepts during his final season at Ohio State. The same outside-zone scheme concept that has made the previous no-name running backs fantasy darlings in the 49ers offense. I doubt we see Sermon open the season as the starter in front of Raheem Mostert, but the speedy 29-year old can only hope to hold off the rookie. However, once Sermon gets churning, I think he will force the 49ers' hand. As the featured back during Ohio State's final three games, Sermon rushed for 640 yards (9.0 yards per carry) and flashed elusiveness with 28 forced missed tackles (30% missed tackle rate). One of Sermon's biggest knocks coming out of school was work in the passing game, but that might not matter considering the team's QB of the future, Trey Lance, won't be checking down too often due to his mobility. If Mostert falters in any way, expect Sermon to take over sooner rather than later.

10. **Michael Carter, NYJ:** The Jets added running back Michael Carter early on Day 3, which destroys any fantasy value for last year's fourth-round pick, La'Mical Perine. The new staff has no ties to him, so the backfield will most likely lean on Carter and Tevin Coleman until the latter indefinitely gets hurt. Carter might not see a workhorse role with the Jets like many are hoping, but I like his upside as a receiver. He's also an explosive runner — he led the nation in 2020 in carries of 15 yards or more — which will hopefully set him apart from a much older Coleman. I fully expect Carter to become the team's No. 1A runner because he fits the outside-zone run scheme so perfectly. Carter finished second last season in PFF rushing grade (87.2) when rushing from outside zone concepts. We also saw him out-rush teammate Javonte Williams in 2020, and some regard Williams as the class' best running back. Additionally, with Carter's explosive upside and pass-catching chops, he gets the nod as the favorite to be Gang Green's RB1 in 2021. That role may never entail 20-plus touches per game, but targets alone will supplement his fantasy value.

11. **Zack Moss, BUF:** Zack Moss was one of the few younger running backs to see his fantasy draft stock rise after the 2021 NFL Draft as he appears to be in the driver's seat to emerge as the RB1 in the Bills backfield. Moss averaged 11.1 fantasy points per game in the eight games he saw double-digit touches last season. We want pieces of high-powered offenses, and Moss is a cheap part of the Bills' offense. Starting running backs can be difficult to come by in the middle rounds. Still, the ambiguity of the Buffalo backfield has made Moss a value as one of the latest potential starters being selected. If he can stay healthy, I think we see a drastically different player in Year 2. He was PFF's second-highest graded pass-blocker among the 2020 rookie class, which bodes well for him continuing to see snaps on third downs. Just be wary of his demanding early-season schedule. With three tough matchups against Pittsburgh, Miami, and the Football Team (all top-13 run-defenses in 2020) followed by three-plus

matchups against Houston, Kansas City, and Tennessee, Moss seems destined to be a late-bloomer in 2021. So just be patient, and reap the rewards when it matters most.

MATCHUP PLAYS

1. **Ke'Shawn Vaughn, TB:** Did we all just completely forget that Bruce Arians called the Ke'Shawn Vaughn "breakout" just a few months ago? Of course, I'm being facetious because Arians constantly makes statements that have zero semblance of the truth to them. We can't take anything Arians says at face value. Still, the second-year pro might have a shot to compete for reps during training camp — an opportunity he didn't get during last year's "offseason" activities. Last year, there were reports that Vaughn was being used as a special teamer. Any suggestion of a role in the offense is a step in the right direction. Leonard Fournette, Ronald Jones II, and Giovani Bernard will all be free agents after the 2021 season, leaving the Bucs' 2020 third-round pick as the only running back on the roster in 2022. With a lack of depth at the position heading into 2022, the Buccaneers could have drafted a running back in the NFL Draft. But general manager Jason Licht did not add to the position, leaving Vaughn's door of opportunity open. It would make sense for the second-year player to see more work so the Buccaneers can fully evaluate what they have in him. The masses are going head over heels for the likes of rookies Michael Carter (107th) and Trey Sermon (88th) but are overlooking the fact that Vaughn (76th) has higher draft capital than *both* of them. Vaughn possesses a three-down skill set and showed in the NFL that his coaches could call on him to pass protect. On 26 total pass-blocking snaps, he earned a PFF pass-blocking grade of 84.3. That ranked second only to Nick Chubb (91.4) among running backs. Conversely, Fournette saw the most pass-blocking snaps (84) among Tampa RBs and was atrocious. His PFF pass-blocking grade ranked 41st out of 42 qualifying running backs. Bernard's addition creates a hurdle to receiving work in the Bucs' backfield, but the newly acquired scatback isn't a lock to seize a massive role on offense, despite what Arians might tell us. His one-year deal with the Bucs is worth less than $1.5 million — nearly identical to the amount of money they paid veteran LeSean McCoy in 2020. As we all know, McCoy was a bust and played a minimal role in the offense. Vaughn out-carried McCoy 31 to 10. Last season, a Tampa Bay RB posted a top-30 PPR performance 15 times. There's fantasy value to be had even in this ambiguous backfield — chasing after the cheapest/overlooked option is the best buy-low option. Vaughn's sunk value has reached a point where there's nowhere to go but up.

2. **Jamaal Williams, DET**: Jamaal Williams is a great value — he's probably going to get more work than anybody invested long-term in De'Andre Swift would care to admit. Lions beat reporters have said Swift could end up being the 1A to Williams' 1B in the backfield. Considering where new head coach Dan Campbell and offensive coordinator Anthony Lynn draw their coaching roots (offenses where the true RB1 wasn't an every-snap player, i.e., Alvin Kamara and Austin Ekeler), Williams could have a role similar to Melvin Gordon III/Latavius Murray. The former Packer played well enough to keep Aaron Jones from seizing an 80% snap share and possesses a three-down skill set that would translate should Swift miss any games. In addition, he is a capable pass-catcher and has also shown that he can be called upon when needed in a larger capacity. During Weeks 7 and 8 last season, with Jones sidelined, Williams averaged 18.8 fantasy points per game and 21.4 expected fantasy points per game. Williams has a sneaky chance to be involved heavily from the get-go with overall talent devoid in the Lions' offense. Detroit's "biting kneecaps" mentality screams they will go full-on operation ground and pound as frequently as possible.

3. **James Conner, ARI:** James Conner entered the 2020 season with aspirations of functioning as a low-end RB1 but failed to deliver. The Steelers running back has been trying to live up to his insane 2018 campaign when he averaged 21.5 fantasy points per game (seventh) but has been unsuccessful thus far. Conner's fantasy points per game have fallen from 14.8 in 2019 (17th) and bottomed out last season at 12.7 (28th). He's not on the right trajectory for NFL teams/fantasy managers to invest heavily in his services. What mediocre fantasy value Conner mustered last season was tied to his 200-plus total touches. That seems like a long shot to repeat with his new team, the Arizona Cardinals. Conner's long-documented history of injuries also makes it severely unlikely we ever see him reach true bell-cow status again. What's more likely to happen in the desert is for Conner to split time with Chase Edmonds, but the former might have the edge over the incumbent in attaining the role at the goal line. Seventy percent of Arizona's carries

inside the 5-yard line are available, which presents a golden opportunity for Conner. Over the past two seasons, Edmonds has only one goal-line carry. Since 2018, Conner has 32. The days of Conner being a locked-and-loaded RB stud are over, but should he carve out a role as an early-down grinder with touchdown upside, he'll deliver usable fantasy weeks.

4. **Kenyan Drake, LV:** Based on hype and draft capital last summer, Kenyan Drake was a big disappointment in fantasy football. He was being drafted as the RB10 overall but finished the year as RB15. In reality, Drake's performance was much less helpful for fantasy purposes, as he finished 27th in fantasy points per game (12.9). The once heavily touted fantasy back ended the season with a 60.9 overall PFF grade, the lowest mark of his career, and averaged only 2.5 yards after contact per attempt. That ranked dead last among all running backs with at least 150 carries. Drake caught 25 passes on 29 targets last season, operating behind Chase Edmonds, the team's primary pass-catching back. Drake served as the team's early-down grinder and wasn't asked to do as much as a receiver. Still, Drake might have been miscast in his role as the early-down back commanding 230-plus carries. He never exceeded more than 170 carries in the previous three seasons and instead was used much more as a receiver. His lackluster season forced him out of Arizona to find a new home with the Las Vegas Raiders. The amount of money shelled out to Drake (the league's 15th highest-paid RB) makes it highly likely this backfield is much more of a one-two punch than Jacobs functioning as a legitimate RB1. With Jacobs almost certainly maintaining his role in early-downs, Drake is a solid bet to see a massive bump in pass-game work and snaps on third down. From 2017-2019, Drake finished 12th overall in targets among running backs, averaging nearly 60 targets per season. He could also earn some carries near the goal-line, which would be a disaster for Jacobs' fantasy value. Drake had 22 carries inside the 5-yard line last season (one more than Jacobs). Drake also dealt with numerous injuries before and during the regular season last year, so using him in a more complimentary/lighter role — or "joker," as Jon Gruden likes to call it — could help his efficiency. One way or another, the ex-Cardinals running back will be involved way more than any Jacobs manager would like. That makes Jacobs a much more difficult running back to select in the third round of fantasy football drafts. At the same time, Drake's arrival in Las Vegas makes him an intriguing and potentially sneaky value several rounds later. The Raiders have the league's most difficult schedule based on forecasted win totals, especially early on in the season. This could force them to play catch up frequently, which will provide ample opportunity for Drake to get peppered with underneath targets from Captain Checkdown, Derek Carr.

5. **Tony Pollard, DAL:** Tony Pollard has been nothing short of fantastic in his limited action in the NFL and possesses league-winning upside should anything happen to Ezekiel Elliott. Since entering the league in 2019, Pollard ranks first in missed tackle rate per attempt (25%) and yards after contact per attempt (4.0) and fourth in missed tackle rate per touch (25%). He's tied with Nick Chubb for the highest missed tackle rate on rushing attempts and tied with Derrick Henry in yards after contact per attempt. Talk about an elite company. We also saw Pollard as the fill-in starter for Zeke in Week 15 against the 49ers, and he did not disappoint. He scored 33 fantasy points — more than any point total Elliott put up all season. Zeke better not miss any more time in 2021, or we might see a new RB1 in Dallas. After Week 13, Pollard earned a 40-plus percent snap share in every single game. Before that time, he played exactly zero games with that sizable workload—stock up for Pollard. Whether Pollard gets his chance at the starting role due to an injury or more touches based on how well he has played, he's got untapped potential worth stashing onto rosters.

6. **Gus Edwards, BAL:** Since the start of 2018, Gus Edwards ranks fifth in PFF rushing grade (90.2) and fifth in yards per attempt (5.1). He doesn't quite have the elusiveness or pass-catching chops like Tony Pollard, but he has a clearly defined role for the Baltimore Ravens. Edwards didn't see fewer than seven carries in a game after Week 13. He also was only slightly out-touched by J.K. Dobbins (74 to 86) during that time. There aren't many other No.2 running backs in the league that will come close to averaging north of ten touches per game. Let alone one that is also as efficient on the ground as Edwards is. His opportunities in the Baltimore offense aren't going anywhere in 2021. They will only expand should anything happen to Dobbins. Behind the top two on the depth chart, there isn't much.

7. **Ronald Jones, TB:** From Weeks 1-14, RoJo was PFF's fifth-highest-graded running back (82.8), and he ranked fifth in yards after contact per attempt (3.6), fourth overall in rushing yards (900), and 13th in fantasy points scored (190.3). He was well on his way to hitting the coveted 1,000-yard mark but dealt

with injuries and COVID to close out the season. The addition of Leonard Fournette right before the season threw a wrench in Jones' fantasy outlook, but all it did was lower Jones' price in drafts. He functioned as the clear early-down back until "Playoff Lenny" emerged, and he should be the favorite to reprise that role even with Fournette back in the fold for 2021. Jones won't be a reliable pass-catcher anytime soon — the lowest receiving grade (29.6) among 58 qualifiers in 2020 — but that doesn't mean he can't have decent fantasy value playing in this offense. In 11 games last season, a Tampa Bay running back posted a top-24 PPR performance. In eight of those 11 (73%) games, a Bucs running back posted a top-15 PPR performance. Drafting Jones is a great way to unearth fantasy value towards the later rounds. He's easily the best early-down back in the Tampa backfield.

8. **A.J. Dillon, GB:** During this offseason, A.J. Dillon would have indeed ended up in the 'Up and Coming' tier. But lo and behold, Aaron Jones ended up re-signing with the Packers, regulating Dillon to backup duties. The second-year back now faces a massive uphill battle to become a significant contributor to the Packers' backfield in 2020. However, he will have opportunities based on the team's history of using a two-back system, and we could see him inherit Jamaal Williams' role. Green Bay passed to the running back position on 22% of their pass attempts in 2020 (sixth-most), so seeing Dillon's role as receiver rise next season is firmly within his range of outcomes. But even so, it's easy to envision Dillon eventually carving himself out a potential role at some point during the season. At 6-foot and 250 pounds, Dillon has the requisite size to be the thunder to Jones' lightning. It also remains to be seen whether the financial investment in Jones will change the veteran's role. It would make sense to retain his usual 60-70% snap share to keep from overworking him. With no other RB of consequence, the team would likely turn to Dillon, who showed promise on limited opportunities (55 carries) last season. He earned an 80.7 PFF rushing grade (80.7, 15th), averaged 5.2 yards per attempt (sixth), 3.4 yards after contact per attempt (seventh), and led the league in missed tackles forced per attempt (31%) in 2020. We saw the potential Dillon possesses in Week 16 versus the Tennessee Titans. It was the only game he saw 20-plus carries, and he totaled 123 rushing yards, with 93 coming after contact. In addition, he forced nine missed tackles in that game alone, which placed him in elite company as one of seven running backs to achieve that feat in a single game during the 2020 season. Should anything happen to Jones, fantasy managers can turn confidently to Dillon as a healthy alternative plan with the expectations set at RB2 fantasy production.

9. **Javian Hawkins, ATL:** Louisville's Javian Hawkins went undrafted, but signed as an UDFA with the Falcons after a highly productive college career. He posted a solid 25% dominator rating over his career and a 30% rating in his second season as a starter. He's a home-run hitter, but apparently, NFL teams were more concerned about his more diminutive stature (5-foot-8 and 183 pounds). Hawkins also offers the one ability that Mike Davis does not possess: explosiveness. Hawkins posted the league's third-lowest breakaway run percentage (15%) in 2020 (min. 150 carries). Arthur Smith's offenses relied heavily on zone concepts in Tennessee, which plays into Hawkins' strengths. He rushed for nearly 800 yards (fourth-best in the class) from strictly zone concepts last season. Many other rookie RBs are buried on depth charts, but Hawkins looks to be just one injury away from busting out. Look for him to impress big time in the preseason. He's got talent and reportedly fell in the draft because of off-field issues.

Chapter 6

WIDE RECEIVERS

Michael F. Florio

PPR SCORING

WR1 PPR		RPV
1	Davante Adams	16%
2	Stefon Diggs	12%
3	Tyreek Hill	9%
4	DeAndre Hopkins	7%
5	A.J. Brown	4%
6	D.K. Metcalf	-3%
7	Calvin Ridley	-3%
8	Justin Jefferson	-3%
9	Keenan Allen	-5%
10	Julio Jones	-10%
11	Allen Robinson II	-10%
12	Terry McLaurin	-12%

WR2 PPR		RPV
1	CeeDee Lamb	5%
2	Amari Cooper	5%
3	Diontae Johnson	5%
4	Adam Thielen	2%
5	Robert Woods	2%
6	D.J. Moore	0%
7	Tee Higgins	0%
8	Ja'Marr Chase	-2%
9	Chris Godwin	-2%
10	Mike Evans	-4%
11	JuJu Smith-Schuster	-6%
12	Odell Beckham Jr.	-6%

WR3 PPR		RPV
1	Brandon Aiyuk	3%
2	Cooper Kupp	3%
3	Tyler Lockett	3%
4	Jerry Jeudy	1%
5	Kenny Golladay	1%
6	Courtland Sutton	1%
7	Robby Anderson	1%
8	DeVonta Smith	-1%
9	Antonio Brown	-1%
10	D.J. Chark Jr.	-3%
11	Chase Claypool	-3%
12	Tyler Boyd	-6%

WR4 PPR		RPV
1	Will Fuller V	8%
2	Brandin Cooks	8%
3	Jarvis Landry	5%
4	Michael Gallup	5%
5	Mike Williams	2%
6	Marvin Jones Jr.	0%
7	Curtis Samuel	-3%
8	Laviska Shenault Jr.	-3%
9	Marquise Brown	-3%
10	T.Y. Hilton	-3%
11	Deebo Samuel	-8%
12	Michael Thomas	-8%

WR5 PPR		RPV
1	Jaylen Waddle	15%
2	Corey Davis	11%
3	Darnell Mooney	8%
4	Rashod Bateman	5%
5	Nelson Agholor	2%
6	DeVante Parker	-2%
7	Cole Beasley	-2%
8	Michael Pittman Jr.	-5%
9	Russell Gage	-6%
10	Gabriel Davis	-6%
11	John Brown	-8%
12	Mecole Hardman	-12%

****See Page 3 for information on how to get RPV Cheat Sheets for one-time fee with free updates in July and August after one time purchase***

STANDARD SCORING

	WR1 STND	RPV			WR2 STND	RPV			WR3 STND	RPV
1	Davante Adams	21%		1	Terry McLaurin	6%		1	Kenny Golladay	4%
2	Tyreek Hill	19%		2	CeeDee Lamb	4%		2	Tyler Lockett	4%
3	Stefon Diggs	16%		3	Adam Thielen	4%		3	Brandon Aiyuk	4%
4	DeAndre Hopkins	3%		4	Robert Woods	3%		4	Cooper Kupp	3%
5	A.J. Brown	3%		5	Mike Evans	1%		5	Chase Claypool	1%
6	D.K. Metcalf	-3%		6	Chris Godwin	0%		6	Courtland Sutton	2%
7	Justin Jefferson	-5%		7	D.J. Moore	-1%		7	D.J. Chark Jr.	0%
8	Calvin Ridley	-8%		8	Diontae Johnson	-2%		8	Robby Anderson	-1%
9	Julio Jones	-9%		9	Tee Higgins	-2%		9	Jerry Jeudy	-2%
10	Amari Cooper	-10%		10	JuJu Smith-Schuster	-3%		10	Will Fuller V	-2%
11	Keenan Allen	-13%		11	Ja'Marr Chase	-4%		11	DeVonta Smith	-6%
12	Allen Robinson II	-13%		12	Odell Beckham Jr.	-6%		12	Antonio Brown	-7%

	WR4 STND	RPV			WR5 STND	RPV
1	Mike Williams	6%		1	Deebo Samuel	7%
2	Brandin Cooks	4%		2	Laviska Shenault Jr.	5%
3	Marvin Jones Jr.	3%		3	Michael Pittman Jr.	3%
4	Curtis Samuel	2%		4	Mecole Hardman	2%
5	Marquise Brown	2%		5	Nelson Agholor	1%
6	Tyler Boyd	1%		6	DeVante Parker	-1%
7	Michael Gallup	1%		7	Darnell Mooney	-2%
8	Jarvis Landry	0%		8	John Brown	-3%
9	T.Y. Hilton	-2%		9	Gabriel Davis	-3%
10	Jaylen Waddle	-4%		10	Russell Gage	-3%
11	Corey Davis	-5%		11	Jamison Crowder	-3%
12	Michael Thomas	-7%		12	Cole Beasley	-3%

Wide receiver is the deepest position in fantasy football. The first two rounds will be littered with running backs, which means if you want to land two of the elite receivers, you likely can in most drafts. But, the receivers available in the fourth and fifth round are so strong that you can wait on the position until then to draft your first receiver and still be fine with who you draft. From those rounds on, the receivers available are better than the options at the other positions (besides QB), which also makes waiting to address the position a possibility. Typically, after you draft your first two receivers, you should be focusing on players that come with upside rather than those who come with just a safe floor.

THE ELITE

1. **Davante Adams, GB:** Adams scored 30 more fantasy points than any other receiver in PPR leagues, and he did so in only 14 games. He averaged 25.6 fantasy PPG, while no other receiver even put up 22 per game. He ranked in the Top-5 among all receivers in yards (1,374), targets (149), receptions (115), and had a league-high 18 touchdowns. He also led receivers with a 30 percent target share, a 37 percent red-zone target share, with 0.81 fantasy points per route run. All of that means that Adams is a beast. He was head and shoulders the best fantasy WR in 2020, but he has been super consistent for years now - scoring at least 16 fantasy points in 83 percent of his games since 2018. The only knock on him is he's failed to play 16 games in four straight seasons. With Aaron Rodgers returning and the Packers still not adding a receiver, Adams should be the first WR off the board in the middle of the first round.

2. **Tyreek Hill, KC:** Hill had his best season to date, finishing as the WR2 in PPR leagues. He has finished as a Top-5 WR in fantasy PPG in three of the last four seasons now. Hill averaged 21.93 fantasy PPG in 2020, the second-most among WRs and one of just two to average over 21 points per game. He scored over 15 fantasy points in 12 games, which was tied for the most by any receiver. He also scored 17 touchdowns while topping 14 in two of his last three seasons. Hill is the ideal combination that you want in a fantasy receiver: he plays in a pass-first offense with a great play-caller, is tied to a great QB, can score fantasy points in chunks due to his downfield ability and as a solid red-zone option. He is an easy Top-5 receiver in fantasy and will be the second receiver off the board in most drafts.

3. **Stefon Diggs, BUF:** When Diggs was traded to the Bills, the belief was that he would help Josh Allen. He certainly did, but Allen also helped unlock Diggs full abilities too. Last season he put up a career-high in fantasy points (328.6) and fantasy PPG (20.54) while leading the league in catches (127) and receiving yards (1,535). No other receiver topped 1,410 yards. He also chipped in eight touchdowns. In 2020, Diggs was one of just two receivers with over 115 catches and 1,400 yards (DeAndre Hopkins). Diggs returns to a very favorable situation as Brian Daboll will still be calling plays, and Allen will still throw him the ball. He is still clearly the Bills' top option after leading them in targets, catches, yards, and receiving TDs last season. He is one of the elite receiver options and will be one of the first four drafted - I would recommend third.

4. **A.J. Brown, TEN:** Brown finished last season as the WR12 in total points, but he was the WR6 in fantasy PPG. He missed two games due to a knee injury that Brown said should have ended his season, but it required surgery after the season. The knee did not slow him down as he posted 1,075 receiving yards and 11 touchdowns. Despite missing two games, he scored over 20 fantasy points in seven games, the third most among receivers. He also finished as a Top-10 fantasy WR in 36 percent of his games, the sixth most among wideouts. Those who had Brown were happy last year, but it was frustrating that the Titans did not throw him the ball more. He did not have a double-digit target game until Week 17 when most fantasy seasons are over. Brown can only learn from the great Julio Jones and although Jones may take away some volume, Brown's calling card has always been efficiency. Also, with a new OC in town, it could just lead to more passing than we have grown accustomed to seeing in Nashville. Brown is a WR1 with sky-high upside.

5. **DeAndre Hopkins, ARI:** Hopkins finished fourth among receivers in total fantasy points and was the WR5 in fantasy PPG. He has finished in the Top-5 in each category in four straight seasons and five of his past six. There were concerns if his targets, or production, would decrease with the move to Arizona, but all he did was top 150 targets for a sixth straight season. That is tied with Antonio Brown for the longest streak in NFL history. His 29 percent target share was second among all receivers. He also topped 1,100 receiving

yards in four straight seasons - the only player in the NFL to do so. He showed that even with the Cardinals, he belongs in the elite tier of receivers, especially if Kyler Murray lives up to the extremely high ceiling he possesses. But some negatives came with the move to the desert. In 2020 he posted a career-low 9.1 air yards per target, and his six touchdowns were his fewest since 2016 - although his touchdowns have decreased in three straight seasons. While he is still in the elite group, he should be the last of this bunch to get drafted.

TOP TALENT

1. **Calvin Ridley, ATL:** Ridley finished as a Top-5 fantasy wide receiver in total points and fantasy PPG in 2020. He racked up 143 targets (9.5 per game), which was a career-high. He did benefit from the absence of Julio Jones last season. In games without Jones, he averaged 11.3 targets per game, 109.2 receiving yards, and 20.56 fantasy PPG. Those numbers dropped to 8.0 targets when Jones was active, 76.1 receiving yards, and 17.45 fantasy PPG. With Jones gone this season, Ridley is taking over as the number one option with the Falcons, just like Jones did with Roddy White 10 years ago. Ridley remains an explosive WR1 option.

2. **Keenan Allen, LAC:** Allen was a clear benefactor playing with Justin Herbert last season. He finished with a 24 percent target share, but it was 29 percent in games with Herbert where Allen did not get injured. He averaged 10.7 targets per game with Herbert and 18.57 fantasy PPG, both of which are better than his career numbers with other QBs. Allen also scored over 20 fantasy points in seven games in 2020, which is even more impressive since he missed two games and was hampered in others due to injury. He finished as the WR7 in fantasy PPG, his third finish as a Top-8 WR in that format in the last four years. He has topped 135 targets in four straight years, the second-longest streak in the NFL, and has reeled in over 100 catches in three of the last four seasons - and had 97 in that other season. He always brought such a safe floor, but now playing with Herbert, his upside is the highest it's ever been. He was putting up Top-5 WR numbers before a late-season injury. Due to that injury, he will not go off the board as a Top-5 WR but take advantage of that and draft him as a WR1.

3. **Justin Jefferson, MIN:** Jefferson exploded on the scene with 274.2 fantasy points, the sixth most among all receivers in 2020 and the fourth most ever scored by a rookie wideout. He finished with 1,400 receiving yards, the most ever by a rookie. Only Stefon Diggs and DeAndre Hopkins had more last season. Jefferson did so in the strangest year ever for rookies, one with no preseason games. He showed that he is a WR1 for fantasy and his team, posting a 26 percent target share, while his teammate Adam Thielen was at 22 percent. There is no reason to believe that Jefferson cannot build off his dominant rookie season. The first-round pick should even command more targets, as his target share grew as the season went on. Initially, it was Thielen they were throwing the most too. He is a WR1 once again for fantasy purposes.

4. **DK Metcalf, SEA:** Metcalf is one of the best athletes in the NFL, and it has translated to fantasy success. Last season he put up the seventh-most fantasy points among receivers (271.3) while showing that he can be exactly what we hoped he would: a great threat downfield and in the red zone. Last season he averaged 11 air yards per game and saw 38 percent of his team's air yards, both ranking in the top-3 among wideouts. He also was in the top three in the NFL with 14 end zone targets and is one of just two players (Mike Evans) to have at least 14 endzone targets in the last two seasons. While there are some concerns about Seattle running the ball more, Metcalf can overcome that because he gains points in such big chunks. He is a WR1 in fantasy because he comes with a safe floor and one of the highest ceilings in the league.

5. **Michael Thomas, NO:** *(Update: Michael Thomas will be missing at least the first month of the season which significantly impacts his re-draft value. Even barring a setback, QB play could further suppress this once former first round fantasy pick)* Michael Thomas had a record-setting 2019 but was largely unavailable due to injury in 2020. But you can give Thomas a pass for that, as he was a Top-10 fantasy WR since he entered the NFL, up until last year. But Thomas comes with more risk this season than ever before as he will have a new QB - and both bring new concerns. If Jameis Winston is the starting QB, he has a history of being more of a downfield thrower, but not as accurately as Drew Brees. And him being a

downfield thrower does not play into Thomas' strengths. If Taysom Hill starts, you have to worry about the Saints running the ball more, especially in the red zone. But, Hill has been an accurate QB in his small sample as an NFL QB. He had a higher adjusted completion percentage in starts over the past five seasons than both Winston and Brees - but again in a small sample size. Thomas is still in the low-end QB1 mix, but his floor and ceiling are lower than in recent seasons.

6. **Terry McLaurin, WAS:** McLaurin has a chance to live up to that Scary Terry nickname this season. Washington went out and signed Ryan Fitzpatrick, who is expected to start for them, which means great things for McLaurin. First, McLaurin is one of the best downfield receivers in the league. He had 34 percent of Washington's air yards last year, the sixth-most in the NFL. Yet, he was doing so with a trio of QBs that have all averaged under seven air yards per attempt. His numbers especially took a hit with Alex Smith, who averaged 5.1 air yards per throw. Fitzpatrick has averaged 8.9 or higher in four of the last five seasons, including over 10 in 2018. He has notoriously peppered his number one receivers with targets, dating back to his days with Stevie Johnson. A high volume of targets plus a QB that can take advantage of his downfield prowess is the perfect combination for McLaurin to be a WR1, with Top-5 upside this season.

7. **Allen Robinson, CHI:** When ARob entered free agency, many wanted him to leave Chicago and land a QB upgrade. But, him staying in Chicago was likely his safest bet at another 150 targets. He is, in fact, one of just two receivers with at least 150 targets in two straight seasons (DeAndre Hopkins), and in each of those seasons, he finished as a Top-9 fantasy receiver. He did so with Mitch Trubisky and Nick Foles in those seasons. Now he will be playing with Justin Fields (Andy Dalton won't hold him off for long), which could be the QB upgrade we had hoped for Robinson. Throughout his career, Robinson has been a WR1 despite never playing with much QB help, but that could change as Fields might be the best QB he has ever played with. Due to the offense he plays in, his ceiling is limited, but there is no reason he cannot repeat as a WR1 for a third straight season.

8. **CeeDee Lamb, DAL:** Lamb is a great breakout candidate heading into the 2021 season. Last year in five games with Dak Prescott, Lamb was averaging 7.8 targets, 88.6 yards, and 17.12 fantasy points per game. Those numbers dropped to 6.4 targets, 45.6 yards, and 11.65 fantasy PPG without Prescott. But those great numbers he posted with Dak came in Lamb's first five career games in a season with no preseason games. Imagine what he could have done had Prescott stayed healthy. Additionally, he lines up in the slot, which provides him with high percentage targets and allows him to take advantage of his great ability to add yards after the catch. Plus, the Cowboys raved all last summer about Lamb's abilities in the red zone, and then he went out and tied for the most end zone targets on the Cowboys (9). In the endzone is an area where teammate Amari Cooper also tends to struggle. So Lamb has a real chance to break out as a WR1, much like Calvin Ridley and Chris Godwin have done in recent years.

9. **Julio Jones, TEN:** Jones has been an elite fantasy receiver for years, but this is shaping up to be the first year in a while that he is not one of the first receivers off the board. Last year Jones played just nine games, as a hamstring injury hampered him. He averaged 85.7 yards per game, which was his fewest in any season since 2012. He averaged 0.51 fantasy points per route run in 2020, on par with his 0.50 in 2019, but decreased from the 0.55+ he posted in the three prior seasons. We know that Jones brings a Top-5 WR ceiling, but there is a very competent WR1 opposite of him, and Jones is a 32-year-old receiver coming off a season hampered by a hamstring injury. Due to that, he will go off the board as a borderline WR1/2. He would be a great pick in the late third, early fourth round of drafts and may have a chip on his shoulder with something to prove now after Falcons dealt him to the Titans in June.

10. **Chris Godwin, TB:** After a breakout 2019 season, Godwin came into 2020 with WR1 expectations and failed to live up to those due to injuries. Godwin only played 12 games in 2020, but he could not live up to the lofty numbers he put up the year before when he was out there. He went from putting up 19.72 fantasy PPG to 15.92. He saw a decrease in his targets, catches, and yards per game as well. He could be better this season as he was limited by injuries in 2020, a strange year where reps were more vital than ever, especially with a new QB. He could be the top weapon for the Bucs again this season, especially given Tom Brady's fondness for the slot. But there are so many options in the passing and rushing game that he could be up and down each week. He should be valued as a fantasy WR2 in around the fourth round of drafts.

11. **Robert Woods, LAR:** Woods has been a consistent WR2 ever since joining the Rams. He has finished as a Top-14 fantasy WR in three straight seasons. He averaged over 15 fantasy PPG in each of those seasons and racked up at least 86 catches. But his receiving yards did drop to 936 this season, his fewest since 2017. He was able to mitigate the fantasy hit by scoring a career-high eight touchdowns in 2020. Still, he has more upside this season, like all the Rams do, after they went out and traded for Matthew Stafford. Woods can make for an especially nice pairing with Stafford since Stafford put up better numbers on play-action passes, while Woods already led the Rams in targets, catches, yards, and TDs on play-action throws. Woods should again go off the board as a WR2, but his ceiling is higher now than in past years with Jared Goff.

12. **Tee Higgins, CIN:** There was a stretch of the 2020 season where Higgins looked no worse than a WR2 for fantasy purposes. From Weeks 3 through 11, he averaged 8.1 targets, 74.3 receiving yards, and 15.53 fantasy PPG. What is the significance of those weeks? Week 3 was when Higgins was injected into the starting lineup, and Week 11 was Joe Burrow's final game of the season. The wheels did fall off a bit after Burrow got injured, but it happened across the board in Cincy, not just to Higgins. Plus, he was able to put up those numbers in perhaps the strangest year ever for rookies. They cast A.J. Green aside to ensure Higgins would get his run, and it paid off for anyone who took a chance on him in fantasy. The only concern is the addition of Ja'Marr Chase, but in both seasons with Zac Taylor, the Bengals ran three WR sets on over 75 percent of their plays. Chase puts a lid on Higgins' ceiling, but he should still be a strong fantasy contributor. He will go off the board as a fringe WR2/3 this season.

13. **Mike Evans, TB:** Mike Evans is the only player in NFL history to top 1,000 receiving yards in each of their first seven seasons. He has also finished as a Top-15 fantasy WR in three straight seasons. Evans was able to produce like usual because he found the end zone 13 times, but it's worth noting that he posted a career-low in targets (109) and receiving yards per game (62.9). His numbers also took a hit when Chris Godwin was active. There are many options once again in Tampa, and if TD regression comes for Evans (and Tom Brady, who threw the second-most TDs of his career), he could struggle to produce Top-15 WR numbers. He will go off the board as a WR2 but could struggle for weekly consistency given the surplus of options in Tampa.

14. **Amari Cooper, DAL:** For years, Cooper had a reputation as a boom-or-bust receiver who would either explode and give you huge production or leave you scratching your head and wondering what happened to your WR1. But last year, he was the opposite - he was more consistent than ever but did not have the huge Cooper game we have become accustomed to. Cooper has now finished as a Top-15 fantasy WR in two straight seasons and Top-21 in five of his six NFL seasons. But Cooper was putting up big-time numbers with Dak Prescott, averaging 11.0 targets, 84.8 receiving yards, and 17.84 fantasy PPG with Prescott. Those numbers fell to 6.8 targets, 62.7 yards, and 13.42 fantasy PPG without Prescott. He is a safe WR2 in this high-powered offense and could flirt with WR1 status.

15. **DJ Moore, CAR:** Moore is one of the more polarizing players in fantasy football. There is no denying his talent, but last year, talent did not lead to a ton of fantasy production. All three of the Panthers' top wideouts (Robby Anderson, Curtis Samuel) averaged somewhere between 14.01 and 14.14 fantasy PPG, with Moore scoring the fewest fantasy points of the trio. Moore, though has finished as a Top-25 fantasy WR and topped 1,200 scrimmage yards in two straight seasons. With Curtis Samuel no longer playing in Carolina, it helps open more opportunities for Moore, but there is a QB change that we will have to worry about. Moore is going off the board as a low-end WR2. That means that you can draft him around where he has finished the past two seasons, but he has the upside to finish higher.

16. **Kenny Golladay, NYG:** Kenny Golladay had a lost 2020 season, playing just five games and finishing with just 338 yards and two touchdowns. But, in each of the two prior seasons, he put up over 1,000 yards. His best season came in 2019 when he had 65 catches for 1,190 yards, 11 touchdowns, and averaged a career-high 15.5 fantasy PPG. Now playing with the Giants, Golladay will need to rely on Daniel Jones to get the ball downfield and in tight windows as Golladay has never been much of a separator but more of a contested-catch specialist. His presence helps Jones and the Giants more than they help Golladay. He is a borderline WR2 for fantasy and may struggle to find weekly consistency.

17. **Diontae Johnson, PIT:** Johnson was the best fantasy receiver on a crowded Steelers team. He led the team in targets, receiving yards, and fantasy PPG. I often joked last season that if Diontae Johnson finished a game, he would lead the Steelers in targets. He did so in the game he was benched for drops!

The Steelers offense is set to run similarly to 2020 when the game plan was to get the ball out of Big Ben's hands as soon as possible, often throwing short to intermediate throws, which only benefits Johnson. He should be a WR2 in drafts and the first Steelers receiver off the board.

18. **Cooper Kupp, LAR:** Kupp is coming off of a down 2020 season in which he caught a career-low three touchdowns and finishing as a WR3 in fantasy. But, if you rostered Kupp last year, you know the end-of-season numbers look even better, considering he had 35 percent of his year-long targets and fantasy points in just three games. But before 2020, Kupp had been a Top-15 fantasy WR in PPG in two straight seasons and finished as the overall WR4 in 2019. The QB upgrade to Stafford should help Kupp as Stafford will air out the ball more. Kupp will get drafted as a borderline WR2/3 in fantasy drafts, but we know he has a higher upside evident by seasons before 2020 when the Rams got away from the pass and became more of a run-first team.

SOLID OPTIONS

1. **Adam Thielen, MIN:** Thielen finished as a WR1 in 2020 largely because of his career-high 14 receiving touchdowns. That made up for the fact that he had just 74 catches and 925 yards. That is far off from what we have come to expect from Thielen - who posted at least 91 catches and 1,275 yards in his last two healthy seasons. Part of what ate into Thielen's numbers was Justin Jefferson blossoming into a true WR1 and seeing a larger target share and simply being the more productive option. I would not bank on another 14 touchdowns to push Thielen up, but he should be valued as a safe-floor WR2 in a Minnesota offense that will lock in on their top targets.

2. **Brandon Aiyuk, SF**: Aiyuk finished 2020 as a WR3 in total points, he was a WR2 in fantasy PPG (15.38), but he broke out and looked like a WR1 down the stretch - scoring over 17 fantasy points in six of the final seven games. He was the WR4 averaging over 18 fantasy PPG in weeks seven on. However, that was mainly with George Kittle and Deebo Samuel out of the lineup. Aiyuk may also have to deal with a new QB as the Niners took Trey Lance third overall, and he could push to start right away. Lance has a strong arm, but he does come with some accuracy issues, and he is an amazing runner who could naturally lead the Niners to pass less. Aiyuk is going off the board as a WR2, which comes with a high ceiling and not the safest floors.

3. **Will Fuller V, MIA:** Fuller was putting up WR1 numbers in 2020 until his season came to a screeching halt when he was suspended six games - serving five last year and the first week of 2021. Look, we know the deal with Will Fuller by this point of his career. He is an excellent field stretcher who will create plenty of separation. Last season in just 11 games, he put up a career-high in targets (75), yards (879), and touchdowns (8). He could top those numbers this year as the number one option in Miami, but it is worth pointing out that Tua Tagovailoa is not the deep ball passer that Deshaun Watson is. As a result, Fuller is likely to have some big games and some dud weeks, depending on the Dolphins game script. He is a great best ball pick, but he is a strong WR3 who has a higher ceiling and comes with some health concerns in redraft.

4. **Odell Beckham Jr., CLE:** Beckham tore his ACL in Week 7 last season but seems to be on track to be ready for the start of the NFL season. Managers will have to monitor OBJ this summer. But he has not been the same receiver for the Browns that he was for the Giants. In 2019, his lone full season for the Browns, he put up 1,035 yards on 74 catches. Last season, he put up 319 yards in his six healthy games - good for an 851-yard 16-game pace. That is not what you expect from OBJ. The Browns will continue to be a run-first offense, meaning we no longer can value OBJ like we used to, as he will not be a weekly star. But he will still have productive weeks, putting him in that high-end WR3 range.

5. **Tyler Lockett, SEA:** Lockett had a career year in 2020, and most fantasy players were left unhappy. He went out and put up a career-high in fantasy points, fantasy PPG, targets, and catches and missed out on a high in yards by just four. But the issue was how inconsistent he was in 2020. Lockett scored 46 percent of his fantasy points (PPR) in just three games last season. He had eight of his ten touchdowns in these three games and over 90 yards in each of them - in the other 13 games, he topped 70 yards just once. If you had Lockett last season, you know how frustrating the end of the season was. Despite being a WR1 at year's end, I would feel much more comfortable drafting Lockett as a high-end WR3 this season.

6. **Courtland Sutton, DEN:** One of the breakout stars of the 2019 season had his 2020 cut short when he tore his ACL in Week 2. He is on track to be ready for the start of the regular season, but you should monitor his health throughout the summer. He not only led Denver receivers in pretty much every category in 2019, but he was Top-8 in the NFL in catches of 20-plus air yards (11), red-zone targets (18), end zone targets (12), and most importantly, he led the league in end zone catches (6). He is both a great deep threat and red/end zone target - the two best ways for receivers to rack up points quickly. He will also have a better QB situation, as the Broncos now have Drew Lock and Teddy Bridgewater, which is a better backup plan than in recent seasons. He is an upside WR3.

7. **JuJu Smith-Schuster, PIT:** While he is included in the WR section, JuJu was used as a tight end would be for the Steelers last season. Last season Smith-Schuster posted a career-low of 5.8 air yards per target. His previous low was 8.9. He also posted a career-low in yards after the catch per reception at 4.22 - his previous low was 5.45. So, not only were his targets shorter than ever, but he was gaining fewer yards after the catch than ever before. He finished as a low-end WR2 last season because he had 97 catches and nine touchdowns, not because of his 831 yards. This season, JJSS will go off the board as a WR3, but with all the same pieces in place in Pittsburgh, he is more of a safe floor, low ceiling option with a better running back. So, he could see those TDs drop off a bit as well this season. It depends on what kind of drafter you are: JuJu is a player for you if you want safety. But if you like the upside in your WR3, you can do better.

8. **DJ Chark Jr., JAX:** Chark let down in 2020, missing time due to injury and just not being nearly as effective as he was in 2019 when he was on the field. It's hard to blame Chark as the Jags turned to Garner Minshew, Jake Luton, and Mike Glennon at QB in 2019 - but he will get a big upgrade in Trevor Lawrence this season. Chark projects to be the number one WR for Lawrence, with Laviska Shenault Jr. and Marvin Jones Jr. rounding out the starting wideouts. Chark is a strong downfield threat and can be utilized in the red zone. Last season he was being drafted as a WR2, but he is going in early drafts as a WR3 and now has the best QB he has ever played with. He is a great upside pick in that range.

9. **Tyler Boyd, CIN:** Last year was a tale of two seasons for Boyd. He averaged 8.7 targets, 6.9 catches, 71 yards, and 16.18 fantasy PPG with Joe Burrow, but those numbers decreased dramatically when Burrow went down. Without Burrow, he posted just 4.6 targets, 2.0 catches, 26.2 yards, and just 6.04 fantasy PPG. He now has more target competition than in recent seasons, with Ja'Marr Chase and Tee Higgins manning the outside and Boyd in the slot. Chase and Higgins are the better downfield options and the superior options in the red zone. Boyd will present a safe target for Burrow, and that is exactly what he will be for fantasy - a safe WR3. He comes with a safe floor but the lowest ceiling of these three Bengals wide receivers.

10. **Robby Anderson, CAR:** Anderson was the latest player to get freed from Adam Gase and find new relevancy in fantasy. Anderson had a career year in his first season in Carolina, posting his first 1,000-yard season, with 95 catches and a career-high in fantasy points (224.1) and fantasy PPG (14.01). Anderson had a 26 percent target share last season, which led all Panthers receivers. He will have a new QB throwing him the ball in Sam Darnold, but his career 1,341 yards, and 11 touchdowns from Darnold are the most any receiver has from the young QB in his career. It is safe to say they have rapport, and with Curtis Samuel now out of town, the volume should be safe for Anderson. Despite all that, he is still going in the WR3 range, well after Moore goes off the board. At that cost, he not only comes with a safe chance of returning that investment, but his deep play ability gives him a higher ceiling as well.

11. **Deebo Samuel, SF:** Samuel looked like a breakout star in 2019, but injuries derailed last season. Samuel only played seven games, and he did not take a step forward when he was on the field. As a result, his fantasy PPG was lower in 2020 (11.53) than it was in 2019 (12.61). Brandon Aiyuk stepped up in his absence, and George Kittle will be this team's top target if healthy. That leaves Samuel and Aiyuk competing to be the second target on an offense that will likely run a good amount, especially once Trey Lance takes over. Samuel will not be asked to be a field stretcher as much as he will be used on short to intermediate passes that allow him to do what he does best - run with the ball in his hands. He goes off the board in the low-end WR3 or high-end WR4 range in early drafts. He will return that value as long as he stays healthy, making him a safe pick, but his ceiling is lower than others that go off the board in that range.

12. **Brandin Cooks, HOU:** After a down 2019 season, Cooks returned to his usual productive self, posting over 1,000 yards for the fifth time in six years. His 15.47 fantasy PPG was the second-most of his career. His 23 percent target share last season was a career-high, while his 81 catches were the second most of his established career. With Will Fuller now playing in Miami, Cooks is the unquestioned WR1 in Houston. But for fantasy, he is simply going off the board as a WR4 - and largely not because of him at all. Cooks comes with many question marks, such as - who will be his QB in 2021? With Deshaun Watson's future both legally and with the Texans so up in the air, it is hard to draft Cooks earlier. He could have a combination of Tyrod Taylor or Davis Mills throwing him the ball - without a lot of offensive help around him. Cooks is about as boom or bust as they come in 2021.

13. **Marquise Brown, BAL:** Brown started the 2020 season with 101 receiving yards, his most of any game last season. It was looking great for those who took a chance on him, but then he scored double-digit fantasy points just two more times through Week 11. But after five weeks of single-digit fantasy points, including a week without a catch, Brown ascended late in the season. From Week 12 through 17, Brown put up 15.97 fantasy PPG, scoring over 12 in every game. He averaged 4.3 receptions, 56.3 yards per game, and scored six touchdowns in that span. The breakout took longer than expected, but it happened. But before you get too excited for Brown, know that the Ravens drafted Rashod Bateman in the first round. Bateman projects to be the x wide receiver on this team, the traditional number one wideout. Brown will be the field stretcher on the opposite side and get used in the slot at times. He will now have Bateman, Mark Andrews, and Sammy Watkins to compete for targets on a team that has thrown the fewest since Lamar Jackson has taken over. Perhaps Baltimore will throw more this season, but given that there is more target competition than ever, Brown is a weekly boom-or-bust WR4 for fantasy purposes.

RED FLAGS

1. **A.J. Green, ARI:** Green was a dominant force for years, but now he is more of a name than a useful fantasy piece. Last season Green played 16 games for the first time since 2017, but he finished 68th among wideouts in fantasy points, and 92nd in fantasy PPG and routinely was shut out as he was cast aside for Tee Higgins. Green missed all of 2019 and played ten games or fewer in two of the prior three seasons, so trusting him to be healthy is a challenge in itself. He could see a resurgence in Arizona, but his last dominant fantasy season came way back in 2016. Green is just a late-round pick at this point in his career, but do not fall victim to drafting a name. There are dart throws that come with much more upside than Green.

2. **T.Y. Hilton, IND:** Hilton was able to stay healthy last season, but it did not lead to fantasy points. It did the exact opposite as he had a career-low in fantasy PPG and total fantasy points (besides injured seasons). His 6.2 targets per game were the fewest he has seen since 2012. Hilton was elite with Andrew Luck and serviceable with other QBs. He will have a new starting QB in 2021, this time with Carson Wentz leading the Colts. He can still be a nice field stretcher that dictates defensive attention at this point in his career, but expecting him to return to anywhere near his old self would be a mistake. He finished as a WR4 last year, but he will be turning 32 this season and relies on speed. That is a deadly combination, and you would be better-suited taking upside shots on other receivers in his range.

3. **Emmanuel Sanders, BUF:** Sanders seems to be outdueling father time, but at 34 years old, he is far from the explosive receiver he once was. Last season was his fewest catches and yards since 2017. Do not see the name and think he will put up big numbers with Josh Allen and the Bills' pass-heavy offense. He will see time, as the Bills ran four-wide receiver sets the second most in the NFL last year (15 percent), and could do so more this season, but when they go three-wide, he may hit the bench in favor of Gabriel Davis. He provides the Bills with a reliable option and some veteran presence, but he is likely a better real-life piece than fantasy. Let someone else draft him.

4. **Sammy Watkins, BAL:** For some reason, fantasy players have a tough time quitting Sammy Watkins. He could not become a reliable fantasy asset with Patrick Mahomes and the Chiefs - there is no way you can trust him with the Ravens and their run-first offense. No team has run more than the Ravens since Lamar

Jackson became the starter. Plus, he is likely behind Mark Andrews, Rashod Bateman, and Marquise Brown for targets. So do not fall for the name anymore.

UP AND COMING

1. **Ja'Marr Chase, CIN:** Chase is reunited with his LSU quarterback in Joe Burrow. The duo teamed up for that special 2019 season where they were part of maybe the greatest offense in college football history. Justin Jefferson gets a ton of hype, and we saw why last year, but it was Chase that was their top wideout in 2019. That season he put up 84 catches for 1,780 yards and a whopping 20 TDs. Chase recorded 46 explosive receiving plays (15+ yards) in 2019, the most among all college receivers. No other player even had 40. He averaged 21 yards per catch, forced 22 missed tackles, and had 16 catches on 33 contested targets. He put up 3.42 yards per route run in 2019 while reeling in 90 percent of his catchable targets and 49 percent of his contested ones. The talent is undeniable. The only question is the amount of work he will see in year one, as the Bengals have Tee Higgins and Tyler Boyd. However, Chase has an already established connection with Burrow and should be drafted in the WR3 range. He has the highest ceiling of the three receivers here.

2. **Chase Claypool, PIT:** Chase Claypool was the epitome of boom-or-bust as a rookie in 2020. He scored over 15 PPR fantasy points seven times, the same number of games he was held in single digits. He scored 20 percent of his fantasy points in one game. But he did show that he is one of the best field stretchers in the league, posting a 30 percent air yard share, the highest on Pittsburgh. He will once again be their deep threat this season, but he will be paired with Ben Roethlisberger and his post-surgery elbow throwing him the ball. Last season Roethlisberger averaged just 6.9 air yards per pass attempt, which ranked 34th of the 44 QBs who threw 100 passes in 2020. But he did average 4.5 passes of 20-plus air yards per game, which ranked 12th. Those deep shots will primarily go to Claypool, and the weeks he catches them will be great for fantasy. He is a borderline WR3/4 with a high ceiling but a somewhat volatile floor for fantasy.

3. **Michael Pittman Jr., IND:** Pittman did not produce enough to be fantasy relevant as a rookie, but he brings a lot of upside coming into 2021. He can play out wide, and in the slot, he can be a downfield threat, although he profiles more like the Colts' top possession receiver and chain-mover. With T.Y. Hilton getting up there in age, the Colts will need someone to step up opposite him, and Pittman has the best chance of doing so. Wentz threw out wide on 34 percent of his throws last season, where Pittman ran 75 percent of his routes. He goes off the board as a WR4 but has a chance to exceed that cost.

4. **Laviska Shenault Jr., JAX:** Is massively popular with the fantasy community, but it could lead to being over-drafted. He goes in the low-end WR3 or high-end WR4 range in early drafts, and he could live up to that, but there have been some worrisome signs from new head coach Urban Meyer. First, he made it known that they were dead set on taking Kadarius Toney because he can be used all over the field, including out of the backfield. Then they drafted Travis Etienne, and they have discussed how he can be used in many creative ways all over the field. That is exactly the role that fantasy hopefuls have pegged for Shenault, but, he did finish strong last season, as the WR16 in the final five weeks of the NFL season. He scored four touchdowns in his final six games after scoring just one in his first nine games. Shenault has DJ Chark Jr. and Marvin Jones Jr. to compete with targets and not a whole lot behind them. Shenault should see enough volume to warrant him being a WR4, but if the hype pulls him up any higher, you can let someone else draft him.

5. **DeVonta Smith, PHI:** Smith takes a lot of heat for his weight, but it should be nearly as large of a factor as it gets made out to be. His weight detractors will point to him getting beat by press coverage, which is when a corner plays close to the line of scrimmage and tries to jam a receiver, but Smith is so good at winning at the line of scrimmage that it was never an issue for him in college. Unlike any receiver we have seen before, Smith can bend and cut almost like he is made of elastic and uses his long wingspan to high point the ball. He is also a complete gym rat. He is like the Kevin Durant of receivers, which is fitting

because he shares the Slim Reaper nickname with him. Oh, and he put up absolute ridiculous numbers at Alabama last year, winning the Heisman. He put up 1,878 yards. No other receiver topped 1,220 yards. He also led the class in yards after the catch with 962; no one else had 660. He also led them with 301 receiving yards after contact. Smith led the class with 23 receiving TDs, 84 first downs, and 44 explosive plays (15+ yards). And he finished third in yards per route run with 4.20 and in contested catches with 12. He is one of the top two rookie wide receivers and should be drafted as a WR3 with upside.

6. **Jaylen Waddle, MIA:** Waddle is a speedster who can play both out wide and in the slot. He was limited to only six games in 2020 but did put up 591 yards and four touchdowns. He did showcase his deep ball abilities, though, averaging 21.1 yards per catch. That's what he did his entire college career, as he averaged at least 17 yards per catch in all three seasons. Waddle picked up 282 yards after the catch, picked up 22 first downs, and had 15 explosive plays (15+ yards) in his limited six games of action. His 10.1 YAC per catch ranked third among wideouts in this class. Waddle also averaged 4.19 yards per route ran, which ranked fourth in this class, just one spot behind former teammate DeVonta Smith. He will now compete with Will Fuller, DeVante Parker, and Mike Gesicki for targets. There are suddenly many weapons in Miami, although they all pretty much come with some injury concerns, which could open a path for more volume. He should be valued as a WR4 with upside, but his weekly production could be very up and down. Nevertheless, he is a strong best ball pick because of his speed.

7. **Jerry Jeudy, DEN:** Jeudy was of the consensus top-two wide receivers in the 2020 draft class. A year later, you would be hard-pressed to put him in the top-two still. But, Jeudy still comes with a lot of upside. Last season he did lead the Broncos in targets (113), targets from Drew Lock (93), and in air yards per game (96). He had two big games where he topped 25 fantasy points, but that equated to 33 percent of his yearly points, as he scored less than 15 in every other week. The Broncos did add Teddy Bridgewater, which could be viewed as a QB upgrade over Lock, but still leaves much to be desired. Jeudy has the talent, and there is no denying that, but the QB play, along with the fact that Courtland Sutton and Noah Fant will see a good amount of targets as well, makes Jeudy too volatile to draft as a starting fantasy receiver. He is better suited as a bench receiver, who we know brings upside.

8. **Darnell Mooney, CHI:** Mooney was up and down as a fantasy asset last season, but he stepped up as the Bears' clear second receiver. He scored double-digit fantasy points in five games last season. But he was second on the Bears in targets per game (6.1) and target share (16 percent), as well as air yards per game (72). His 23 targets of 20-plus air yards led the Bears last season. He will never be the Bears' top target, as Allen Robinson has that on lock, but Justin Fields is a QB upgrade, especially on deep balls. Mooney should be valued as a boom-or-bust reserve wide receiver in drafts, but he does have fantasy upside if he can become a more consistent option with Fields. He is a nice best ball pick as he will have some big weeks when he connects on the long ball.

9. **Rashod Bateman, BAL:** Bateman ended up going to the Ravens, who have thrown the fewest in the NFL since Lamar Jackson took over. Last season they threw on a league-low 44 percent of plays (only the Patriots were also below 50 percent), and in 2019 that number was also 44 percent (no other team was below 51 percent). That number could increase this season as the Ravens made adding pass-catchers a priority this offseason. Bateman gives Jackson a receiver as he has never had before - one that can win contested catches and not just rely on creating separation. He is also an explosive option as he had 11 explosive pass plays (15+ yards), which may not seem like much compared to the others, but he played just five games due to a shortened season and had 36 catches. That means 11 of those 36 catches, or nearly a third, went for over 15 yards. In that limited 2020, he caught 36 balls for 472 yards and two TDs. His best college season was in 2019, when he posted 1,219 yards and 11 TDs on 60 catches as a sophomore. He averaged a ridiculous 20.3 yards per catch that season. He still managed over 13 yards per catch in each of his other two college seasons. Bateman should be valued as a WR4 with upside in 2021 redrafts, but he is the Ravens receiver you should most be interested in (sorry, Marquise).

10. **Terrace Marshall Jr., CAR:** On paper, it is easy to think of Marshall as the Curtis Samuel replacement, but he gives Carolina a weapon they have lacked in recent years. Marshall was one of the best contested-catch prospects in this class. He's 6-foot-two and used that size to win contested targets at an 82 percent clip this past season. That was the highest percent of any player that had at least seven percent of their targets contested. In addition, he showed his downfield abilities with 15.2 yards per catch and had 15 catches of at least 15 yards. Marshall will be behind Christian McCaffrey, DJ Moore, and Robby Anderson

in the target pecking order, but there is a real chance he leads this team in red/end zone targets. He is a reserve wide receiver for fantasy purposes in 2021, but he does have upside and really could blossom into a must-start option as soon as 2022.

11. **Rondale Moore, ARI:** Moore landed in a great spot with Kyler Murray and the Cardinals. He is expected to play in the slot, where Murray threw 31 percent of his passes last season. Moore's best college season came as a freshman when he went off for 114 catches for 1,258 yards and 12 TDs while adding in 213 yards and two TDs on the ground. He was limited by injuries in 2019 and a reduced 2020 season since. In that big 2018 season, he ran 694 routes in the slot and just 52 out wide. He will compete with Christian Kirk for slot routes, but the Cards do run four-wide receiver sets more than any team in the NFL - 20 percent in 2020. That will naturally lead to Moore getting snaps, but he will have to beat out Kirk, or have an injury, to get enough snaps to be fantasy relevant. Moore, like many of the rookie receivers, comes with upside but not the safest of floors. He should be drafted as a reserve receiver in the double-digit rounds of redraft leagues.

12. **Amon-Ra St. Brown, DET:** St. Brown, who is the younger brother of Packers receiver Equanimeous and the son of a former bodybuilding world champion, fell to the fourth round, but he also fell into one of the best fantasy landing spots. The Lions receiving core is thin. St. Brown will compete with Breshad Perriman, Tyrell Williams, Quintez Cephus, and Kalif Raymond for receiver targets. Not only is it thin, but those other receivers project more as out wide and downfield receivers, while St. Brown can slide in and provide Jared Goff with a big, athletic slot receiver. I am trying to say that he could be Goff's new Cooper Kupp, albeit not as good. There is a chance for him to lead this receiving group in targets in year one, and he is one of the better late-round gambles to take at the receiver position.

13. **Kadarius Toney, NYG:** Toney is a freak athlete who is the most dangerous receiver in this draft class after the catch. But, he is still raw as he only made a move to receiver in college, and his route running needs work. He put up 984 yards and 10 TDs on 70 catches in the passing game. He rushed for nearly 600 yards in his college career as well. He picked up 27 explosive plays (15+ yards) and forced 20 missed tackles, both of which ranked in the top-five in this class. Toney could be a useful weapon, but he did not fall into the best landing spot to unleash him in year one. First, the Giants have many targets in Kenny Golladay, Sterling Shepard, Darius Slayton, Evan Engram, and Saquon Barkley. The other is that Jason Garrett is not the most creative play-caller. Toney has upside, but he likely will be inconsistent. He is a late-round pick that is better suited for best ball in year one.

14. **Elijah Moore, NYJ:** Despite the shortened 2020 season, Elijah Moore had a career year. He went off for a college career-high 86 catches, 1,193 yards, and eight touchdowns in just eight games. He went in the early second round of the NFL Draft to the Jets, expecting that he would play out of the slot and provide Zach Wilson with an explosive target across the middle. He often gets comped to Tyler Lockett, another receiver who is a legit downfield threat out of the slot. Moore should be targeted as a reserve-round receiver, but he comes with upside, especially if the Jets move on from Jamison Crowder. He is a strong best ball pick.

15. **Gabriel Davis, BUF:** Davis was slow to get going out of the gate in 2020, but once John Brown was sidelined due to injury, he received more playing time and came to life in the second half. He caught five touchdowns from Week 9 on and showed out enough that the Bills decided to move on from Brown in the offseason. He will now compete with Emmanuel Sanders for targets behind Stefon Diggs and Cole Beasley, but Davis is both more explosive and better out wide at this point in their careers. He is a reserve round wide receiver with an unsafe floor, but he has breakout potential.

16. **Van Jefferson, LAR:** Robert Woods and Cooper Kupp are getting a lot of hype since the QB upgrade from Jared Goff to Matthew Stafford, and for a good reason. But, neither of those are suited to play the old Brandin Cooks role, which Jefferson could fill. Last season, Jefferson and Josh Reynolds, who will now play in Tennessee, were the only Rams receivers with an aDOT over 9 (both were over 11). The Rams drafted Tutu Atwell and signed DeSean Jackson, showcasing that they want to throw the ball downfield more. One of those three will end up being a late-round value, and I would put Jefferson with the highest odds of those three.

17. **Tutu Atwell, LAR:** Atwell was listed under 150 pounds heading into the NFL draft, but reports are that he's now in the 160s. Still, that is small for an NFL receiver, but he certainly has the speed and shiftiness to be productive. Atwell posted over 800 receiving yards in his last two seasons in college and at least five

touchdowns. He will compete with Van Jefferson and DeSean Jackson to play as the flanker in the Rams infamous three-wide receiver sets. You should monitor that competition all summer, but the expectation is that Atwell will either be a late-round upside flier or an undrafted player that could become a waiver wire target this season.

18. **Mecole Hardman, KC:** With Sammy Watkins now out of town, Hardman has his best shot at being a regular fantasy contributor. Hardman has shown his big-play ability ever since he stepped foot on an NFL field, but the issue has been consistency. Last season he scored over 18 fantasy points twice and over 10 five times - but he had less than 10 in 11 games and less than three in five games. That is not useable in fantasy as you have no idea what he could give you, and the floor is way too low. But that could change this year as the Chiefs need a receiver to step up opposite Tyreek Hill. Hardman's competition for that role is Demarcus Robinson and Byron Pringle. Hardman is a great best ball pick as a WR4 in the 10th round or later, but he should be valued as a reserve receiver with upside for seasonal drafts.

19. **Parris Campbell, IND:** You have likely heard the saying, "the best ability is availability." Being healthy has been Campbell's biggest challenge since entering the NFL. In his two seasons as a pro, he appeared in just nine games, including just two in 2020. We have not seen enough of him at the pro level to say what he will be yet, but there is high potential here. He is a speedy slot receiver who can be a downfield threat. Wentz threw to the slot on 32 percent of his throws in 2020. It is easy to envision Campbell being a strong target for Wentz and the Colts and being a nice fantasy asset if he can stay healthy. He can form a nice receiver trio with Pittman and Hilton, but he is a WR5 that you can target in the late rounds to find some upside for fantasy.

20. **Tre'Quan Smith, NO:** Smith has had a lot of hype in his young career, but he has totaled 1,109 yards and 14 touchdowns in three NFL seasons. He's never topped 500 receiving yards in any season in his career. Smith is a receiver who can line up out wide and be an explosive downfield option. The issue has been that Drew Brees, in his later years, was not the kind of QB to air it out. Instead, he would get the ball out quickly and rely on timing and accuracy with receivers - something Smith has struggled with in his NFL career. But, there is hope for Smith still. If Jameis Winston starts for the Saints, and we will have to monitor that situation all summer, he is a QB that fits Smith's skill set better. He is not afraid to air it out, throw into tight coverage and let his receiver go up and get the ball. If Smith flames out again this year, we can forget about him as a fantasy asset, but he is worthy of a very late-round flier just in case Winston can get the most out of him.

SERVICEABLE WITH UPSIDE

1. **Antonio Brown, TB:** Antonio Brown had six years matched by few in NFL history. But he has played just nine games total the last two seasons due to off-the-field issues. Last season he debuted in Week 9 and got off to a somewhat slow start. But in his final six games, playoffs included, he caught six touchdowns. He can still play and will serve as the third receiver behind Mike Evans and Chris Godwin for Tom Brady. His week-to-week production will likely fluctuate as there are many target options in this offense, but he is always an injury away from seeing a big increase in his weekly target share. He is going as a WR4 in early drafts - which is a fine gamble to take on his upside. Always monitor his off-the-field situation before drafting him.

2. **Marvin Jones Jr., JAX:** Jones continues to produce while being underrated in fantasy. He has finished as a Top-30 wide receiver in fantasy PPG in four straight seasons and the Top-30 in total points in three of the last four seasons (played nine games in the other). Jones is also a strong red-zone presence, scoring nine touchdowns in three of the past four seasons. Jones moved on from Detroit to Jacksonville, where he will team up with DJ Chark Jr. and Laviska Shenault Jr. to form the "ALL Jr." receiving core for Trevor Lawrence. Luckily for them, you can expect Jacksonville to run a lot of three wide receiver sets. In Lawrence's college career with Clemson, they used a three-receiver set on 84 percent of plays, while Urban Meyer used it 76 percent of his time with Ohio State. Jones provides a good downfield weapon and red-zone target. You can draft him as a WR5, but that is a good value as he has a strong chance of being the number two target in a pass-heavy offense. He is especially great in best ball drafts.

3. **Mike Williams, LAC:** Williams is the king of getting hyped up in the preseason and then finishing as a WR4. But, this season, in early drafts, he is going as a WR5. We know what Williams is at this point of his career - he is a strong deep threat and a good red zone option. Philip Rivers was never able to unlock him fully, but a stronger-armed QB like Justin Herbert could. The Chargers also greatly upgraded their offensive line this offseason and lost Hunter Henry, and do not have a lot of WR depth behind Williams and Keenan Allen. Williams could dictate a higher target share than ever before in this offense, and it costs cheaper than ever to acquire him. He is a strong pick as a low-end WR4/high-end WR5 in the double-digit rounds.

4. **Michael Gallup, DAL:** After finishing as a WR2 in 2019, Gallup finished as a WR3 in total points but as a WR5 in points per game. Gallup was the weird Cowboy player that did not see a big dropoff when Dak Prescott was injured. In those first five weeks with Dak, he was the third target behind Amari Cooper and CeeDee Lamb. Gallup averaged 11.56 fantasy PPG, but just 5.6 targets per game with Prescott, but averaged 10.5 fantasy PPG and 7.06 targets per game with the other Cowboys QB. Five games are too small of a sample size to say this is how the targets will be distributed this season, but Gallup likely remains third behind the other two big receivers. But, he will be their best deep threat, meaning that he could put up big numbers on weeks where he connects on a long one. Due to his down 2020, you can draft him as a WR4 in the double-digit rounds. He is a strong best ball option, and a solid upside shot as a reserve receiver as the Cowboys could be the best passing attack in the league this season.

5. **John Brown, LV:** Brown was in and out of the Bills lineup in 2020, only playing nine games and seeing a career-low 52 targets. A year prior, he was a WR2 in fantasy, putting up over 1,000 yards and six scores on 72 catches. He showed the ability to be a field stretcher throughout his entire career and has the possibility of replacing Nelson Agholor in the Raiders' offense. That may not sound like much, but Agholor was a WR3 with nearly 900 yards last season. And you can make the case that Brown is a better deep play receiver than Agholor. His competition for that role and targets behind Darren Waller is Henry Ruggs III. The Raiders have an incentive to get Ruggs more involved after drafting in as the first receiver taken in the 2020 draft, but Jon Gruden is also a coach that loves veterans. Brown is purely a late-round pick, but he can greatly outlive that cost if he takes over that role.

6. **Henry Ruggs III, LV:** The Raiders selected Ruggs as the first receiver overall in the 2020 NFL Draft and then gave him 43 targets on an eight percent target share. It was not a great start to his career, especially given what some other rookie receivers did, but it was one of the strangest NFL seasons in recent history. The Raiders do have the incentive to get Ruggs going in year two, and with Nelson Agholor gone, they will need someone to step up and replace him as both their top receiver and their best field stretcher. Ruggs has blazing speed and will compete with John Brown for that role. He is being drafted as a WR5, sometimes later, in drafts meaning that he is free. You can take a shot on his upside in the late rounds of drafts.

7. **Breshad Perriman, DET:** Perriman showed out with the Bucs at the end of the 2019 season but never got going with the Jets. That is more so on Adam Gase and the 2020 Jets offense, but Perriman is an afterthought in many fantasy drafts because of it. He will once again get a shot as a team's top receiver, this time with the Lions, who have arguably the weakest receiver group in the league. Perriman is still a good deep threat and the most established receiver on the Lions roster. You can get him in the later rounds of the draft, and his weekly volume alone makes it a solid pick.

8. **Jalen Reagor, PHI:** Year one did not go as planned for the first-round wide receiver as he finished the season with just 31 catches for 396 yards and one touchdown. He did show a good downfield threat, as advertised, but he struggled with consistency and dealt with some injuries. Reagor will team up with DeVonta Smith as Jalen Hurts top receivers. Reagor will likely be a deep threat while Smith will play the x. Reagor will probably finish third in target share if everyone stays healthy behind Dallas Goedert and Smith. But, there should be questions about how often Philly will pass this season. Reagor is a boom-or-bust WR5 that is best suited in best ball.

9. **Darius Slayton, NYG:** After a strong rookie campaign, Slayton regressed and finished as a WR5 in fantasy, but he was the WR70 in fantasy PPG. Simply put, he was not usable in fantasy, especially when you factor that his best game of the season came in Week 1. Kenny Golladay is now aboard as the clear-cut number one target, leaving Slayton competing with Sterling Shepard, Evan Engram, Kadarius Toney, and even Saquon Barkley for targets. He provides the Giants with a good downfield and solid red-zone weapon, and since those are the most valuable fantasy targets, he could carve out a nice role. Still, barring injury, he

likely struggles to get enough volume each week to be anything more than a bye week replacement. But he does have upside if any of the Giants receivers, especially Golladay, miss time.

10. **Bryan Edwards, LV:** Edwards had hype coming into the 2020 season but failed to make any impact, totaling less than 200 yards and scoring just one touchdown in Week 17. Still, Edwards showed strong hands and the ability to be a possession receiver who will move the chains in college. The Raiders will be searching for someone to step up, so Edwards will be worth monitoring throughout the preseason. If he has buzz during training camp, he could become a late-round flier to take a shot on.

11. **Sage Surratt, DET:** The Lions receiving core is one of the weakest in the NFL, which means there will be a competition for targets this summer. Surratt did not play in 2020 due to Covid, but in 2019 he put up 66 catches for 1,001 yards and six touchdowns. The lack of playing in 2020 led to him going undrafted in the NFL Draft, but he will have a chance to earn work with the Lions. He is more of a player to monitor this summer who could blossom into a waiver wire pickup during the season.

SERVICEABLE AND SAFE

1. **Corey Davis, NYJ:** After struggling his first three years in the league and looking like a first-round bust, Davis had a career year (so far) in 2020. He put up a career-high in fantasy points, fantasy PPG, yards, and touchdowns while tying his career-high in receptions. Davis finished as both a WR3 in total fantasy points and fantasy PPG. He turned that success into a payday with the Jets. He will now operate as Zach Wilson's WR1, with Denzel Mims, Elijah Moore, Jamison Crowder, and Chris Herndon serving as his primary target competition. He should see safe volume as the likely top target here, but he does come with concerns. The biggest concern is how efficient the Jets offense will be - with a first-time play-caller and rookie QB, this offense naturally could be up and down. Plus, he draws a tough slate of cornerbacks playing in the AFC East. The other concern is Corey Davis a true WR1 in the NFL? He struggled before getting to play second fiddle to A.J. Brown. Due to these concerns, he is a WR4 with a safe floor but not the highest ceiling.

2. **DeVante Parker, MIA:** Parker scored the second-most fantasy points and PPG of his career in 2020, but it was still a significant falloff from his 2019 season. That year he broke out in a big way in the second half of the season and won many fantasy players championships. Last season he had eight games with double-digit fantasy points, but he topped 20 just once. His yards decreased in 2020 by over 400, and his touchdowns decreased by more than half. He also was more productive in games Ryan Fitzpatrick started, but Tua Tagovailoa will be making all the starts (while healthy) in 2021. Plus, Parker has more competition for targets as the Dolphins signed Will Fuller V and drafted Jaylen Waddle in the first round to go along with Mike Gesicki. As a result, Parker should be valued as a WR4 in fantasy. He is best suited as a reserve receiver who you can use in good matchups, but his ceiling is lower than Fuller and Waddle.

3. **Jarvis Landry, CLE:** If you love safe players without a ton of upside, Landy is the player for you! He has finished as a WR3 or higher in each of his NFL seasons, but last year was his worst finish as WR32, and that is in PPR, which is Landry's best format. Last season was his fewest fantasy points scored and scrimmage yards since his rookie season. That was on a Browns team that lost Odell Beckham Jr. in Week 7 and had Austin Hooper in and out of the lineup. The Browns will be a team that relies heavily on their RBs, and when they do pass, Baker Mayfield will not throw to the slot often. In 2020 he threw just 25 percent of his passes to the slot - Matt Ryan and Kirk Cousins were the only regular starters to do so less. Landry, who has notoriously operated out of the slot, ran only half his route from the slot last season. Perhaps he should go inside more since his numbers took a hit. Either way, there is more target competition on a team that wants to rely on their run game. Landry is a safe borderline WR3/4, but he does not come with the highest of ceilings. In non-PPR formats, you should go in another direction.

4. **Cole Beasley, BUF:** Beasley does not bring a high weekly or seasonal ceiling, but he does bring a safe floor. He has scored less than nine fantasy points in his two years with the Bills just six times. He has topped 105 targets in both seasons with the Bills and finished as a WR3 each year. He scored over 15 fantasy points five times last year, three times topping 22. Unfortunately, he does not come with a ton of upside, so he is not a great best ball pick. A reliable 10-points can be great in season-long leagues when dealing with bye

weeks or injuries, but in best ball, that doesn't do a whole lot. Due to the lack of upside, Beasley goes in the WR5 range, which is where he belongs. He will finish higher than that in the Bills' pass-happy offense.

5. **Nelson Agholor, NE:** After an up and down tenure with the Eagles, Agholor went to Vegas and had a career year. He put up 896 yards and eight touchdowns while averaging a by-far career-high 18.7 yards per catch. He turned that year into a payday with the Patriots. He will be their top receiver, but he will have to battle off the tight ends, Jonnu Smith and Hunter Henry, for targets. Much of the passing game will depend on which QB starts for the Patriots, as their styles could not be more different. Cam Newton will lead to a run-first offense, while Mac Jones is not very mobile and will be much more of a pocket passer. Either way, this passing game is not one to get super excited about for fantasy purposes. Agholor is merely a late-round receiver who you should consider in the WR5/6 range, but you should be chasing a higher upside at that point.

6. **Jamison Crowder, NYJ:** Crowder has been a WR3 in the past two seasons and has scored at least 160 PPR points in four straight seasons. He is a reliable slot receiver who does not have a high ceiling but has a safe floor. He is of the same mold as Cole Beasley. Last season he averaged career-high yards per game, but it was only 58.3. Crowder also has competition as the Jets drafted Elijah Moore in the early second round of the NFL Draft, specializing in the slot. In the final year of his contract, Crowder could be a cap casualty if the Jets decide to move on. He is a safe floor receiver (unless cut) and goes in the WR5/6 range. But that deep, you should be taking a shot on receivers with higher upside.

7. **Sterling Shepard, NYG:** Shepherd finished as a WR4 in total points and WR3 in fantasy PGP in 2020. He did so while running just 31 percent of routes from the slot, his career-low. He has recorded 80-plus targets in all five NFL seasons and topped 700 in four of the past five seasons. Last season he had an 18 percent target share, which was the second-highest of his career. The knock on him is he does not score touchdowns. He has scored four touchdowns or fewer in four straight seasons. He is a talented receiver who coaches can move all over the field, which helps his fantasy value as the more you're on the field, the better. But, the Giants receiver room is suddenly crowded. He will have to compete with Kenny Golladay, Darius Slayton, Kadairus Toney, Evan Engram, and Saquon Barkley for targets from Daniel Jones. Shepard was more of a safe floor than a high upside player, to begin with, and the added competition for targets only lowers his floor. He is a late-round pick, but one to avoid and target a player with a higher ceiling.

8. **Russell Gage, ATL:** Gage had a career-high in targets, receptions, yards, touchdowns, fantasy points, and fantasy PPG in 2020 but still was just a WR4. He was able to take advantage of a Falcons offense that suddenly had fewer pass-catching options than usual, and Julio Jones missing time only opened up more work. Jones is now gone, but Ridley is a beast. They added Kyle Pitts to go along with Hayden Hurst, and they signed a pass-catching running back in Mike Davis. Gage is not likely to see the volume he did in 2020, but he may be a worthy of a bench spot and matchup plays.

9. **Tim Patrick, DEN:** Patrick will not see enough volume to warrant being drafted as he will be behind Courtland Sutton, Jerry Jeudy, and Noah Fant for targets on a team that will throw to the RBs as well. Patrick will serve as their primary number three wide receiver, but K.J. Hamler will also get involved. Patrick did put up 742 yards and six touchdowns last season with Sutton out. He is best left on the waiver wire to start the season, but he will become a player to pick up if any injury occurs.

Chapter 7

TIGH ENDS

Derek Brown

PPR SOCRING

TE1 PPR				TE2 PPR		
Player	Proj FPTS	RPV		Player	Proj FPTS	RPV
1 Travis Kelce	355	64%		1 Irv Smith	150	7%
2 Darren Waller	280	29%		2 Cole Kmet	150	7%
3 George Kittle	260	20%		3 Mike Gesicki	150	7%
4 Kyle Pitts	230	6%		4 Evan Engram	145	3%
5 T.J. Hockenson	205	-5%		5 Rob Gronkwoski	140	-1%
6 Mark Andrews	205	-5%		6 Tyler Higbee	140	-1%
7 Dallas Goedert	200	-8%		7 Anthony Firkser	140	-1%
8 Jonnu Smith	195	-10%		8 Jared Cook	140	-1%
9 Noah Fant	180	-17%		9 Hunter Henry	135	-4%
10 Logan Thomas	180	-17%		10 Adam Trautman	135	-4%
11 Robert Tonyan	160	-26%		11 Gerald Everett	135	-4%
12 Blake Jarwin	150	-31%		12 Eric Ebron	130	-8%

STANDARD SCORING

TE1 STND				TE2 STND		
Player	Proj FPTS	RPV		Player	Proj FPTS	RPV
1 Travis Kelce	215	74%		1 Irv Smith	80	20%
2 Darren Waller	165	34%		2 Cole Kmet	80	20%
3 George Kittle	155	26%		3 Jared Cook	80	20%
4 Kyle Pitts	135	9%		4 Mike Gesicki	75	13%
5 Mark Andrews	125	1%		5 Evan Engram	70	5%
6 T.J. Hockenson	120	-3%		6 Rob Gronkwoski	70	5%
7 Jonnu Smith	110	-11%		7 Hunter Henry	65	-3%
8 Dallas Goedert	100	-19%		8 Anthony Firsker	65	-3%
9 Noah Fant	95	-23%		9 Tyler Higbee	55	-18%
10 Logan Thomas	90	-27%		10 Adam Trautman	55	-18%
11 Robert Tonyan	85	-31%		11 Zach Ertz	55	-18%
12 Blake Jarwin	85	-31%		12 Eric Ebron	50	-25%

*****See Page 3 for information on how to get RPV Cheat Sheets for one-time fee with free updates in July and August after one time purchase****

Every year in fantasy football, the late-round tight end options are the talk of the town. Once the season commences, though, the reality always sets in that the tight end position harvests a few select choices. Players like Travis Kelce are weekly difference-makers who give you a statistical advantage and are elite options even compared to other positions. However, once those are gone, the cupboard is filled with hopes, dreams, and thin fantasy options.

My preferred method for attacking the position every season is paying up for the premium difference makers or cobbling together two tight ends with my final picks and playing waiver wire roulette. However, if you can find Logan Thomas-like lightning in a bottle, it can put your team over the top. Additionally, several big uglies exist in the red zone to target fitting a plethora of draft strategies.

THE ELITE

5. **Travis Kelce, KC:** It's nice to be the king, baby. Travis Kelce still reigns supreme as the crowned monarch of the tight end position. Last season Kelce crushed all in his path leading the position in targets (146), receptions (105), receiving yards (1,416), and air yards (1,295). To put Kelce's utter dominance in better context, if you stacked his fantasy points per game (20.9, PPR) up against other positions, he would have finished as the WR3 or RB5. Kelce finished with 0.1 fantasy points per game higher than Derrick Henry. Kelce is the difference maker worth paying up for in drafts. He'll fight Tyreek Hill again for the team lead in targets on an offense that will threaten to lead the league in neutral script passing rate.

6. **Darren Waller, LV:** If Darren Waller played with a quarterback that was even 75% Patrick Mahomes, he would be discussed in the same breath as Kelce. However, Waller is still in his prime, entering his age 29 season, so don't expect him to slow down after last year's meteoric box score excellence. Last year Waller's 28% target share ranked behind Davante Adams, DeAndre Hopkins, and Stefon Diggs among all wideouts and tight ends. In keeping with the Kelce comparisons, Waller was equally impressive and worth the draft capital when sizing his production against other positions. In 2020 Waller would have been the WR8 (PPR) or RB9, which puts him in rarified air. Waller is essentially a discount Kelce that you can draft in many cases 2-3 rounds later.

7. **George Kittle, SF:** George Kittle remains among the elite tier despite some pesky concerns about his ability to stay healthy and his target share this season. Since 2019 Kittle has missed ten games with an injury list consisting of a foot fracture, MCL sprain, hamstring strain, knee sprain, and ankle fracture. Last season Weeks 5-7 was the only stretch of the season where Kittle, Brandon Aiyuk, and Deebo Samuel were all on the field together, playing 62% or higher snaps. In that three-game span, Kittle still garnered a 27% target share and 25% of the air yards. If he can remain healthy and continue to match those numbers, he is deserving of a top-three ranking among the position. The 49ers have ranked 20th, 29th, and 16th in passing attempts over the last three seasons. San Francisco needs to remain at least middle of the pack in passing attempts to have the volume to support Kittle's early ADP. If both of those boxes are checked, Kittle is due for another good top-shelf season.

TOP TALENT

1. **Mark Andrews, BAL:** It's fair to call Mark Andrews' 2020 season a slight letdown after his explosion onto the tight end scene in the previous year. Despite finishing as the TE4 (12.2) last year, Andrews' fantasy points decreased by 1.6 points per game versus the prior season. Last year Andrews finished behind only Darren Waller in target share (25%) at the tight end position. The Ravens infused talent into this passing game with the draft selections of Rashod Bateman and Tylan Wallace. With those additions, Andrews bumps down a peg from elite consideration to an above-average option. Baltimore ranks 32nd (44%) over the last two seasons in neutral script passing rate, so Andrews is likely to feel the sting of more competition for targets. Andrews is still efficient enough to finish inside the top five at the position even with the volume concern, but he'll need a productive year in the touchdown department to do so.

2. **T.J. Hockenson, DET:** T.J. Hockenson enters the season with a fantastic opportunity to improve upon last year's career highs in targets (101) and receiving yards (723). Hockenson's biggest adversary for target

dominance is Detroit's rookie slot receiver Amon-Ra St. Brown. A plus for Hockenson is the Lions' new signal-caller (Jared Goff), who will fall in love with Hockenson's playmaking ability over the middle of the field. Hockenson ranked fourth among all tight ends in yards after the catch (328) and eighth in missed tackles forced (7). Goff ranked 36th in aggressive throw rate last year. As a result, Goff won't shy away from Hockenson running wide open over the middle play after play.

3. **Dallas Goedert, PHI:** Dallas Goedert will still have to contend with the zombie corpse of Zach Ertz if he's still on the roster come Week 1, but there's no disputing he's the number one tight end for Philadelphia now. Goedert showed last season that he's a sure-handed threat at all levels of the field. Last year he ranked seventh in deep targets (9) with a 125.0 passer rating when targeted 20+ yards down the field. Jalen Hurts will pepper last year's sixth-ranked tight end in true catch rate (92.0%). Goedert was the TE10 (10.6) in fantasy points per game last year with Ertz in tow, but if Ertz leaves, Goedert could find himself inside the top five this season.

SOLID OPTIONS

7. **Irv Smith Jr., MIN:** Irv Smith has teased us with his possible upside for the last two seasons. Now with Kyle Rudolph in New York, we could see fully unleashed Irv Smith glory in 2021. Irv Smith missed some time with a back injury last year, but after returning to a full-time role without Rudolph, he flashed this juicy upside. In Weeks 15-17, with Smith playing 79-88% of the snaps, he was the TE11 (11.7, PPR). With only Tyler Conklin to contend with now, Smith assumes the top receiving role on the tight end depth chart for an offense that ran 24.1% of their red-zone passing attack through the tight end position. Smith has a double-digit touchdown upside in 2021.

8. **Logan Thomas, WAS:** Logan Thomas enjoyed a breakout season last year competing with Terry McLaurin for the lead chair in Washington. Thomas led all tight ends in routes run (576), ranked third in targets (110), fifth in deep targets (11), and seventh in red-zone targets (17). Thomas doesn't find himself higher on this list because Ron Rivera and the front office brought in passing weapons this offseason. Last year, he fought for pass game looks with Cam Sims, Isaiah Wright, J.D. McKissic, and Seven Sims. This season Washington will have Curtis Samuel or Adam Humphries lining up in the slot and Dyami Brown running on the outside. Thomas's size (6'6") will keep him active in the red zone, so a top 12 upside is there, but the volume is coming down in 2021.

9. **Noah Fant, DEN:** Noah Fant quietly ended the season as the TE12 (10.0) in fantasy points per game. Unfortunately, nagging injuries kept Fant from actualizing more fantasy output after logging two games with 50% or lower snaps, and he missed another contest. Courtland Sutton's return is concerning to Fant's overall target volume, but he still has the talent profile to weekly duke it out for the second read in the passing game. In 2020 Fant ranked eighth in yards per route run (1.76) and third in yards after the catch (383) among all tight ends. Unless Denver turns into a run-heavy, sluggish offense, Fant should comfortably land inside of the top 12 at the end of the season.

10. **Robert Tonyan, GB:** Robert Tonyan came out of nowhere to finish as the TE6 (11.0) in fantasy points per game last year. Tonyan did this on the back of insane efficiency. In 2020 among all tight ends with 25 or more targets, Tonyan ranked second in catch rate (88.1%), fifth in yards per target (9.93), and first in receiving touchdowns (11, tied with Travis Kelce). That otherworldly type of effectiveness is difficult to repeat ever, much less yearly. The plus for Tonyan is Green Bay has done nothing this offseason to add competition for targets to this passing game. So, any bump in target volume can help him compensate for any backsliding in other categories.

11. **Anthony Firkser, TEN:** Anthony Firkser now finds himself atop a tight end depth chart on a team that finished fourth in the NFL in target share (29.6%) to the position. Firkser will take up the starter's mantle from Jonnu Smith. Make no mistake, when Firkser is on the field, his calling card is as a receiver. Last season he led all tight ends (with 20 or more targets) in slot snap percentage (71.3%), surpassing fellow receiving threats Mike Gesicki and Logan Thomas. Firkser might not be the most athletic tight end in the NFL, but with the lack of quality receiving options around him and the Titans' offensive scheme, he's in line for a ton of volume.

12. **Rob Gronkowski, TB:** Rob Gronkowski defied the masses after a year layoff in his return as a solid fantasy asset. Gronkowski played a full 16 games for the first time since 2011. His weekly availability helped him coast to a TE8 finish in total PPR points (149.3), while his weekly production wasn't as shiny. Gronkowski was the TE16 last season in fantasy points per game (9.3). You could make a straightforward case that Gronkowski is more of a matchup play, but sadly weekly volatility describes the overwhelming majority of the position. He finished with six top 6 finishes at the position last season, so when Brady is in the mood to target the touchdown spike machine, there's a ceiling to be had. Here's to believing that at age 32, he's got one more productive season left in the tank.

RED FLAGS

1. **Mike Gesicki, MIA:** Add Mike Gesicki on top of a growing list of tight ends who will see their roles decrease in the upcoming season because of talent added around them. Gesicki ranked eighth in route participation and targets per snap last season. Gesicki played 67.4% of his snaps from the slot last year as Miami's de facto starting inside receiver. Jaylen Waddle will command that role this year for the Dolphins. Gesicki's blocking skills have never been what has earned him snaps, so Hunter Long could easily play inline over him. Gesicki has gone from the second option in the passing game to a tertiary piece in one offseason.

2. **Evan Engram, NYG:** If we're going to talk target squeeze, Evan Engram's name has to be included as well. The return of Saquon Barkley, the addition of Kenny Golladay, Kyle Rudolph, and Kadarius Toney spells terrible news for Engram. Engram was force-fed targets last season (fourth-most at tight end, 109), but sadly the results were abysmal. Engram ranked 21st in yards per route run (1.34) and had the fourth-highest drop rate (9.2%) at tight end. Engram could lose targets and snaps weekly to Rudolph, who profiles as a better underneath fit for Jason Garrett's offense. The best hope for Engram's 2021 outlook is that the Giants deal him before the season to an offense that will utilize him in the open field again.

3. **Eric Ebron, PIT:** Eric Ebron ranked eighth in targets (91) last year, helping him finish as the TE14 in fantasy points per game (9.5). It's hard to see Ebron even matching that type of production this year. Pittsburgh has a full receiver room returning with Diontae Johnson, Chase Claypool, and Juju Smith-Schuster leading the way. Still, the most considerable dent in Ebron's value is in the backfield. Ebron's made his money since arriving in Steel City with targets over the short middle, but Najee Harris is coming to wreck that in 2021. The Steelers running back target share fell to 32nd (12.8%) in the NFL last year. That number is coming up with Harris running routes as a check-down option. Ebron will likely be a matchup play at best this year.

MATCHUP PLAYS

6. **Jonnu Smith/ Hunter Henry, NE:** If you're drafting either of these players as a weekly set and forget option in your lineups, all I can say is good luck. The Patriots opened up the checkbook after concluding the 2020 season bringing in Henry and Smith along with Kendrick Bourne and Nelson Agholor. The Patriots are a week-to-week game plan-specific team that will feed targets to the easy matchup. This is a beautiful NFL tactic, but for fantasy purposes, it's the stuff of nightmares. Henry and Smith will each have their share of top 10-12 performances, but trying to predict who and where will be an exercise in futility. *(Author's Note: For the record, I believe Jonnu Smith is the going to emerge as a fantasy force despite what my bald brother DBro says here. That is all. ~ Joe)*

7. **Tyler Higbee, LAR:** The hope of Tyler Higbee continuing the season-ending dominance of 2019 into 2020 was crushed weekly by Gerald Everett. Everett was a constant thorn in Higbee's side, cutting into his routes and targets. Now that Everett is out of town, many will gravitate back to Higbee, but concerns persist. Brycen Hopkins and his 76th percentile speed score linger on the roster, as well as fourth-round selection Jacob Harris. Harris is a converted wide receiver who is an athletic marvel. Higbee did manage four top 12 fantasy tight end performances last year, so not all hope is lost. However, he'll be a more

volatile option than some believe because Hopkins or Harris could easily assume a similar role that Everett occupied previously.

8. **Austin Hooper, CLE:** Austin Hooper closed last season with three consecutive top 8 fantasy tight end performances while averaging 8.6 targets per game during that span. Hooper's problem entering this season is Odell Beckham Jr. will be returning to the lineup. During Beckham's seven games played, Hooper surpassed 11 fantasy points only once. In an offense that ranked 28th in pass attempts last year, there's only so much volume to go around, and Beckham will command a large chunk of it. Hooper will log some top 10 fantasy games this year, but they'll be too sporadic to count on him weekly. Hooper is an excellent punt option at the end of drafts if you're grabbing two tight ends and playing the streaming game.

9. **Gerald Everett, SEA:** Gerald Everett reunites in Seattle with his former position coach with the Rams, who is now the Seahawks offensive coordinator. This same coach was in Los Angeles when the Rams selected Everett in the second round of the NFL Draft. Seattle has integrated their tight ends into their passing attack every season before 2020. In the three previous years, Seattle ranked 9th, 11th, and 2nd in target share to TEs, averaging a 29.6% share of the passing offense. Everett will compete with Will Dissly weekly for snaps and targets, but he's got the talent to command the majority share. In addition, Everett has ranked top 12 in each of the last two seasons in reception per broken tackle among all pass-catchers.

WATCH LIST

1. **Blake Jarwin, DAL**: Blake Jarwin is a talented player that we never had the chance to see flourish last season. Jarwin tore his ACL in Week 1, and that was that. Jarwin returns to a loaded passing attack that will compete for the league lead in passing attempts, so volume shouldn't be a significant concern. In a part-time role in 2019, Jarwin ranked sixth in yards per target (8.9) and eighth in yards per route run (2.37) at the position. Jarwin might be the fourth or fifth option in this passing game, but this offense could lead the NFL in points scored, so even a tiny piece of this pie is tasty.

2. **Chris Herndon, NYJ:** Chirs Herndon is a fantastic post-hype sleeper worth monitoring. Herndon is finally free from the crushing clutches of Adam Gase. When Herndon hasn't been on the trainer's table or sidelined by suspension, he's been a matchup nightmare for opposing coordinators to contend with. The Jets' new offensive coordinator helped oversee a passing game in San Francisco over the last three seasons that ranked 5th, 5th, and 10th in target share to the tight end position. Is Herndon George Kittle? Of course not, but he's an athletic mismatch that's flashed when featured. He'll be undrafted in many 12 team leagues and is worth holding over a second quarterback or defense.

UP AND COMING

1. **Kyle Pitts, ATL:** Kyle Pitts flies into a Falcons' offense that led the NFL in passing attempts (626) last season. There's a bevy of passing volume and pass-catchers sharing a field with Pitts that can give him fits for targets. Pitts has to contend with Calvin Ridley, along with Russell Gage and Hayden Hurst. However, with Julio Jones off to the Titans, Pitts now has a target path to cash in on the hype in year one. The rookie tight end transition period is natural, but as we've seen from Pitts collegiate production, he's a unicorn, so it wouldn't be the most shocking occurrence for him to sidestep this trend. Pitts ranked first amongst all collegiate tight ends last year in yards per reception and second in yards per route run against man coverage. Since 2017 Evan Engram is the only rookie tight end to finish a season top-five in fantasy points per game. He did so on the back of 115 targets which were the second most for a rookie tight end since 1992, behind only Jeremy Shockey's 128. Pitts producing top-five numbers is unlikely, but more possible with Julio Jones out of the mix.

2. **Cole Kmet, CHI:** Sadly, Jimmy Graham remains on the Bears roster for now, so Kmet's sky-high ceiling is capped at the moment. That could change at the drop of a hat, though. In Weeks 13-17, Kmet was integrated as a primary piece of the aerial attack. He averaged 27.2 routes per game in that five-game sample with an 18% target share (six targets per game). If Kmet can carve out enough of the red zone

role, then there is a top 12 upside still available for him even with Jimmy Graham in town. Add on top a quarterback upgrade with Justin Fields, and Kmet could be Chicago's Dallas Goedert this season.

3. **Adam Trautman, NO:** The number three option in the New Orleans passing game is up for grabs. Adam Trautman or Tre'Quan Smith could easily stake their claim this year behind Michael Thomas and Alvin Kamara. There will be targets up for grabs if it's Jameis Winston or Taysom Hill throwing them passes. Especially at the tight end position the volume threshold for a top 12 option is low. Because of salary cap turmoil, the Saints were forced to gut their defense this offseason and could be playing catch up quite often this year. Trautman could be a red zone monster for Sean Payton in 2021 with his 95th percentile agility score and 82nd percentile catch radius.

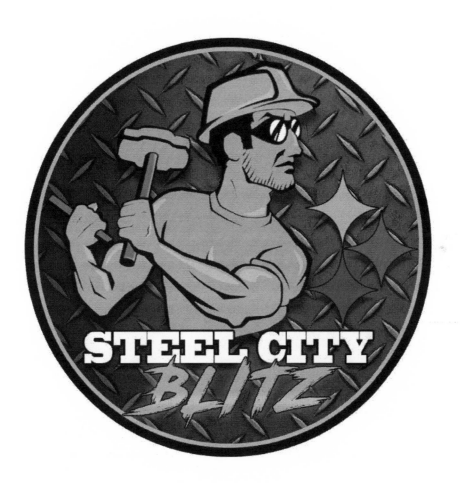

Chapter 8

Kickers

Travis Sumpter

Tier 1

1.	Justin Tucker, BAL
2.	Harrison Butker, KC
3.	Younghoe Koo, ATL

Tier 2

4.	Greg Zuerlein, DAL
5.	Will Lutz, NO
6.	Jason Sanders, MIA
7.	Rodrigo Blankenship, IND
8.	Matt Prater, ARI
9.	Robbie Gould, SF

Tier 3

10.	Tyler Bass, BUF
11.	Jason Meyers, SEA
12.	Marvin Badgley, LAC
13.	Ryan Succop, TB
14.	Mason Crosby, GB
15.	Jake Elliott, PHI
16.	Daniel Carlson, LV
17.	Joey Slye, CAR

Tier 4

18.	Brandon McManus, DEN
19.	Ka'imi Fairbairn, HOU
20.	Chris Boswell, PIT
21.	Dustin Hopkins, WAS
22.	Josh Lambo, JAC
23.	Zane Gonzalez, ARI
24.	Stephen Gostkowski, TEN

Welcome to the stone age! Well, at least if you are an old-school player who enjoys having kickers on your team. Most leagues have gone away from kickers and to me, it is truly a lost art in fantasy. Occasionally, I try to think of ways to make kickers relevant to fantasy leagues again. In my home league The Splash Brothers, we still utilize the kicker position and I truly enjoy the randomness of it all.

If you do play in a league where the kicker is utilized, it is important not to take a kicker too early as you could be passing on some potential breakout stars or even handcuffs late in your draft. If Defenses are already dropping off earlier than expected and you are on the clock in the 14th round and not very many kickers have gone off the board yet; I will take my shot on one of the tier 1 kickers which you can find below.

Stream the position: Otherwise avoiding the position altogether is probably your best option if your league allows it during the draft. Usually at home league drafts or some other apps that allow you to skip the position entirely during the draft is maybe your best option.

When streaming your kickers there are a few different approaches to take in this and are as follows:

1.   Play the waiver wire game. Were there any elite kickers or upcoming matchups that you feel good about that were dropped because of a bye week?

2.   Look at the teams your kicker is going up against. Do they generally give up a lot of points each week and how many red zone opportunities do you believe will be afforded to them? Does the opposing team allow a lot of yards but not a lot of touchdowns?

3.   Watch the weather. Nothing worse than a kicker that is playing against 25-30 mile per hour winds. I prefer my kickers to be playing in a dome or some type of enclosed structure on a given week. Lions, Falcons, Saints, Vikings, Raiders, Cowboys, Texans, Colts, Cardinals, Rams, and Chargers are all stadiums I prefer my kicker to be playing at because they are weathered controlled.

Week 1 Kickers to Stream:

•   Ryan Succop, TB has a very juicy matchup against The Dallas Cowboys defense and should have plenty of red zone opportunities in that match-up. The Dallas defense did do what they could to improve on defense during the draft, but in all honesty, they are not really looking any better off than they were last year.

•   Rodrigo Blankenship, IND versus the Seattle defense in Week 1 and they are not that far from what the Cowboys offer in terms of playing defense. Also, have to kind of a given he might also be a streamer of the week because The Indianapolis Colts also play a home game in that retractable roof stadium.

•   Josh Lambo, JAC The Jaguars take on the lowly Houston Texans team that should be terrible right off the bat. Lambo could see a lot of field goal opportunities in this one as it is also played in a retractable roof stadium. While Lambo is not ranked that high initially it would not surprise me if he finished in the top 12 kickers in 2021. It will be interesting all around to see what Urban Meyers does with this offense as it could be feast or famine.

Experiment: Most leagues make kickers score 1 for Points After Attempt or PAT and 3 for Field Goals or FG. Do what you want to do to keep it fun. In leagues that play with kickers, these are my preferred settings.

1.   1 point for PAT

2.   -1 point for missed PAT

3.   3 points for 1–39-yard FG

4.   4 points for 40–49-yard FG

5.   5 points for 50 yards or more

Chapter 9

TEAM DEFENSE/SPECIAL TEAMS

Derek Brown

The name of the game with defense for our fantasy football leagues is stream. Stream. Stream. Unless your league rules require it, I'll openly advocate for not drafting a defense and instead picking up a DST post-draft before Week 1 and playing the matchups weekly. The scoring margin for defenses inside the top 12 is slim on a weekly basis. While we have numerous metrics to quantify defensive prowess for teams, kick returns for touchdowns, pick-sixes, interceptions, etc., are hard to forecast. The variance is high on any of those outcomes because any cornerback could drop an interception as easily as a returner can get tackled at the one-yard line.

Looking at the last three years of passing defensive data and building upon my previous defensive work for the black book, strong pass defense units have the highest correlation with top 12 fantasy defense finishes. Charting run defense metrics previously from 2016-2019 (Rush defense DVOA, rushing yards per game allowed, and yards per carry allowed), the top 12 finishers in these categories only logged 37.5 to 45.8 percent hit rate. In the 2018-2020 seasons, the top 12 teams with the lowest passer rating allowed held a 72.2% correlation of finishing as a top 12 fantasy defense. This is all to say: Target strong pass defenses and reap the rewards.

Below I'll dive into my Top 24 fantasy football defenses for 2021, outlining enough options to cover 12 team leagues where you will roster two defenses to alternate streaming.

1. **Baltimore Ravens:** Despite losing sack leader Matt Judon and Yannick Ngakoue in the offseason, the Ravens are my top defensive unit this season. Baltimore restocked in the NFL Draft, adding talented pass rusher Jayson Oweh to a defense that ranked fourth in pressure rate (26.8%) last year. The secondary returns Marcus Peters, Marlon Humphrey, and Jimmy Smith after allowing the sixth-fewest passing yards (3,536). Baltimore finished as the DST4 last year but could command the top spot in 2021.

2. **Tampa Bay Buccaneers:** Tampa Bay is in full run-it-back mode returning a stellar defensive unit. The Buccaneers added Joe Tryon in the first round to a defense ranked fourth in sacks (48) and third in pressure rate (27.5%). The secondary hit their stride down the stretch and in the playoffs. Tampa Bay could give the Ravens a run for their money for the top overall spot.

3. **Washington Football Team:** Washington is another top-shelf option led by stud pass rusher Chase Young. Ron Rivera's secondary could be even better this year after allowing the second-fewest passing yards (3,068) and net yards gained per pass attempt (5.3) last year. Adding outside corner William Jackson to start opposite Kendall Fuller was a masterstroke. Teams will have a tough time finding a weakness in this secondary.

4. **Los Angeles Rams:** Aaron Donald and Jalen Ramsey headline a talented defense in Los Angeles. Brandon Staley departs but enters Raheem Morris to direct a squad that finished as the number one DST in fantasy last season. Losing cornerback Troy Hill will hurt, but Darious Williams is still a stud starting with Ramsey. Donald and

Leonard Floyd and their combined 24 sacks return to spearhead a pass rush that ranked second in the NFL in sacks (53) last year.

5. **Cleveland Browns:** The Cleveland Browns could be the most improved defense in the NFL this season and an elite unit. How can a defense ranked 25th in defensive DVOA make this type of leap, you say? Getting full seasons from Denzel Ward and Greedy Williams would be a good start. The additions of Jadeveon Clowney, Troy Hill, Greg Newsome, Jeremiah Owusu-Koramoah, and the return of Grant Delpit (injury) add up to an entirely new defense taking the field in 2021. Clowney upgrades a run defense that allowed the 12th lowest yards per carry (4.3) last year.

6. **New England Patriots:** New England spent the offseason making over a defense that struggled at times in 2020. The Patriots managed to finish 18th in pass defense DVOA but were the worst defense in the NFL against the run last season. Bill Belichick added Henry Anderson, Davon Godchaux, Montravius Adams, and Christian Barmore to upgrade the run-stopping capability. Ronnie Perkins, Matt Judon, and familiar face Kyle Van Noy were brought in to accentuate a pass rush that ranked fifth in pressure rate (26.4%) despite finishing 26th in sacks (24). If Stephon Gilmore has one more season of near-elite production left in him, this defense could be among the league's best again.

7. **Buffalo Bills:** Buffalo did well in retaining their studs on defense by resigning Matt Milano and giving Micah Hyde an extension. Adding a high upside pass rusher like Gregory Rousseau in the draft could pay huge dividends for the aggressive Buffalo front. Last season the Bills ranked eighth in blitz rate (35.8%), so expect defensive coordinator Leslie Frazier to let Rousseau pin his ears back and get after the passer. The Bills were the eighth-ranked fantasy defense last season. If Buffalo gets improved health from Milano and an immediate presence from Rousseau, that could be their floor this year.

8. **Miami Dolphins:** The Dolphins, led by shutdown corners Xavien Howard and Byron Jones, finished sixth in pass defense DVOA last year. Howard and Jones helped Miami tied for the second-most interceptions (18) and second-fewest passing touchdowns (21) in the NFL. Brian Flores dialed up blitz at the second-highest rate (40.8%) behind only the Baltimore Ravens. After the front office added Jaelan Phillips in the draft, expect them to generate more pressure this season.

9. **Kansas City Chiefs:** The Chiefs have finished as a top 12 fantasy defense in each of the last six years and still don't get the respect they deserve. Last year they ranked fifth in interceptions (16) and quarterback knockdowns (66). Chis Jones and Frank Clark return to lead a disruptive pass rush while Tyrann Mathieu creates havoc on the back end. The Kansas City offense gets most of the press, but their defense deserves some love, too, in fantasy football circles.

10. **Denver Broncos:** The Broncos' pass rush was the strength of their defense last season after injuries ravaged the secondary. Bradley Chubb and Von Miller combined for 15.5 sacks in 2020, and if the new look cornerback room can lock down opposing wideouts now, that number will rise. The Broncos wasted no time bringing in Kyle Fuller after the Chicago Bears foolishly decided to cut him. Fuller took away half of the field for Chicago last year, allowing a 55.3% catch rate. He'll team with Ronald Darby and Patrick Surtain II to form one of the best cornerback trios in the NFL.

11.   **Minnesota Vikings:** The 2020 season was a nightmare one for Mike Zimmer and his defense. Michael Pierce (opt-out) and Danielle Hunter (neck injury) missed the entire season, which crushed their defensive line. Hunter and his 29 sacks over the two previous seasons returning will be an absolute game-changer. Cameron Dantzler and Jeff Gladney experienced on-the-job growing pains for their rookie seasons. Dantzler's play picked up down the stretch as he resembled the physical corner the Vikings thought they were getting in the third round of the 2020 draft. Tack on the additions of Patrick Peterson and Xavier Woods to the secondary, and the Vikings are primed for a huge bounce back on the defensive side of the ball.

12.   **Los Angeles Chargers:** Brandon Staley takes over a defense that has the talent to be a top 5-10 unit this year. Joey Bosa leads the pass rush while Linval Joseph clogs the middle, and Derwin James creates problems for opposing passers in the secondary. Asante Samuel is a big upgrade at corner opposite Michael Davis. Staley helped mold a Rams defense that was crushing their opponents weekly last season. The talent is here for him to do the same with the Chargers this season.

13.   **Indianapolis Colts:** The Colts were the third ranked fantasy defense last season finishing behind only the Rams and Steelers. Chris Ballard added Kwity Paye to the pass rush after losing Justin Houston and Denico Autry this offseason. Paye will team with DeForest Buckner to try and improve on last year's 18th finish in pressure rate. The Colts will need Xavier Rhodes to hold off father time for another season if they hope to hold it down on the back end.

14.   **Chicago Bears:** The Bears quietly ranked eighth in defensive DVOA last season. Chicago will need a bounce-back season from Robert Quinn to finish in the top 12 fantasy defenses this year. Quinn disappointed with only 2.0 sacks last year after 11.5 with Dallas in the previous season. The Bears corner situation could also be a problem spot after Jaylon Johnson. Chicago is counting on Desmond Trufant and Artie Burns having anything left in the tank, which are risky bets to make. Overall, the defense has enough top-end talents like Khalil Mack and Roquan Smith to mask some of these deficiencies, but the holes in this defense could become glaring ones easily.

15.   **Pittsburgh Steelers:** The Steelers have Stephon Tuitt and T.J. Watt upfront to bring the heat. The two combined for 26 sacks last season, leading the charge for a defense that led the NFL in pressure rate (35.1%). The concerning aspect of the Steel Curtain is the cornerback room. Steven Nelson is gone, and the team is leaning on Justin Layne, Arthur Maulet, or James Pierre to take the starting spot alongside Joe Haden. Haden can still hold his own, but opposing passing attacks could pick on the other two Pittsburgh starting corners all season long. The pass rush will have to make things hectic for opposing quarterbacks to compensate.

16.   **San Francisco 49ers:** Former NFL linebacker and 49ers linebacker coach DeMeco Ryans steps up to the plate as the new defensive coordinator with the departure of Robert Saleh. Ryans will command a defense ranked seventh in pass DVOA and tenth in rush defense DVOA last year. A defensive line of Arik Armstead, Javon Kinlaw, and Nick Bosa can match up with the best in the league. The secondary will miss Richard Sherman and Akhello Witherspoon, but if Jason Verrett can continue the comeback trail and Emmanuel Moseley can bounce back to his early 2019 form, they'll be just fine.

17.   **Arizona Cardinals:** The Arizona secondary is suspect, but their pass rush will be among the best in the league. Adding Zaven Collins with J.J. Watt and Chandler Jones will give opposing offensive lines a tough assignment weekly. They'll have to because a starting trio of Malcolm Butler, Robert Alford, and Byron Murphy isn't scaring anyone. The Cardinals were eighth in pressure rate (25.9%) and fourth in blitz rate (39.4%) last season. Expect both of those marks to repeat or improve in 2021.

18.   Green Bay Packers: The Packers' defense is a streamer play only. Green Bay fields a better NFL defensive unit than for our purposes in fantasy football. The Packers ranked 18th in total fantasy points last year among defenses. They were 24th in hurry rate and 27th in pressure rate. Jaire Alexander is a premier lockdown corner, but unless you're playing in point-per-shadow coverage leagues, he isn't going to help you much.

19.   New Orleans Saints: The Saints had to slash contracts for the salary cap, and they did so heavily on the defensive side. With Janoris Jenkins, Trey Hendrickson, Sheldon Rankins, and Kwon Alexander all headed out of town. New Orleans is counting on Marcus Davenport to finally become the player they envisioned when taking him in the first round in 2018. Against any soft competition, the Saints can still have some good steaming weeks as Dennis Allen's squad is always looking to create turnovers. Last year New Orleans ranked eighth in offensive drives ending in a turnover.

20.   Carolina Panthers: The additions of A.J. Bouye (if healthy) and Jaycee Horn could be massive for this defense. Youngsters Brian Burns and Jeremy Chin have flashed big-time playmaking ability. Burns rolled up 21 quarterback hits and nine sacks last year. Chin racked up 117 tackles while scoring two defensive touchdowns. If Haason Reddick and Donte Jackson can repeat banner seasons, this defense could surprise in 2021.

21.   Dallas Cowboys: The Cowboys defense has a chance to take a step forward. The question is how much. Dallas ranked 23rd in total defensive DVOA last year. The pass rush will be hit or miss with DeMarcus Lawrence back to lead the squad. Dan Quinn needs Micah Parsons and Kelvin Joseph to hit the ground running and Trevon Diggs to repeat his solid play over the back half of 2020.

22.   New York Giants: The Giants added oft-injured corner Adoree Jackson in the hopes he can lock down the other side of the field opposite James Bradberry. Blake Martinez will again fly around the field, tackling anything in sight. The biggest question is can the Giants repeat their top ten (10th) pressure rate (25.5%) finish from last season. If OLB Azeez Ojulari can be a difference-maker in year one, it's possible.

23.   New York Jets: Robert Saleh has his work cut out for him with this defense. The run defense at least gives him a starting block to begin the marathon. Last year the Jets ranked 8th in run defense DVOA and should be up there again. Quinnen Williams and Sheldon Rankins will clog this middle. The big problem for Saleh is the secondary. Blessuan Austin and Bryce Hall are going to be burnt all year long. These two corners combined to allow a 71.8% catch rate.

24.   Seattle Seahawks: When your sack leader is Jamal Adams, you've probably got a big problem upfront. Adams was exceptional with 9.5 sacks last season, but no other Seattle defensive player had more than Jarran Reed (6.5 sacks). Losing Shaquill Griffin, Jarran Reed, and K.J. Wright is going to sting. With stretch run stops in Houston (if Deshaun Watson is out) and Detroit, Seattle has some streaming appeal in Weeks 14 and 17.

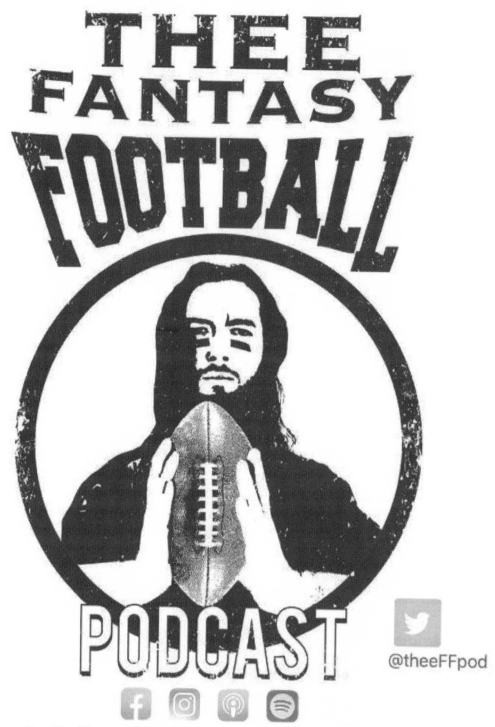

THEE FANTASY FOOTBALL PODCAST

@theeFFpod

Entertaining. Informative. Hilarious.

Chapter 10

IDP

Scott Bogman

Why should I play IDP?

Fantasy Football is better when you can roster players on both sides of the ball. I know you can draft a team defense but it just isn't the same. A team defense is as strong as its weakest link but you don't have to depend on the weakest link if you are picking the players yourself! I also like that IDP takes some of the luck out of Fantasy Football, the more players you have the less likely a freak week or injury is going to sink you. That's from a season level too. If you make some good picks/adds on the defensive side you can push yourself away from the pack or put yourself into the playoff picture. I also feel sometimes, as a person that plays in an absurd amount of leagues, I can get a little one sided in my enjoyment of games. In my opinion there's nothing better than coming back on Monday Night Football because my DB picked off a pass or wracked up 10 tackles. Adding IDP makes the game more fun in my opinion and that's why we all started playing isn't it?

What is standard scoring in IDP?

This is probably the biggest issue in standardizing IDP in most leagues. There isn't really a standard as far as IDP goes. The one that our friendo Gary Davenport and I used for the leagues we ran on *Fantrax last year had the following*:

Solo Tackle - 1.5
Assisted Tackle - 0.75
Sack - 4
INT - 4
Forced Fumble - 2
Fumble Recovery - 2
Pass Defense/Deflected - 1
TD - 6

Yahoo has there own standard scoring:

Solo Tackle - 1
Assisted Tackle - 0.5
Sack - 2
INT - 3
Forced Fumble - 2
Fumble Recovery - 2
Pass Defense/Deflected - 1
TD - 6

This will give you a high-end score of a 15-13ish average for the best LBs, same for DBs and top out around 10 for the best DL. The top end QBs average between 30-25, RBs and WRs just over 20, and TEs are usually around 15. Scoring can be adjusted if your league would like to have both sides of the ball represented equally. I feel like because of the variance in scoring and the unpredictability of IDPs it's better to keep them a little lower than the offensive side but, as stated before, there is no real standard.

When do we need to take IDPs in a draft?

Devin White was the highest scoring IDP last year and his 14.78 average per game made him the 73rd ranked overall scorer in PPR leagues last year. That average would have made him the 33rd in QB scoring, 20th as an RB, 22nd WR and 4th as TE. The 6th round is about the right spot in a 12 man league.

How many IDPs to add

Beginners - 3 total, 1 DL, 1 LB, 1 DB
The "starter set" for IDPs, this lets everyone have a need to focus on all 3 spots and gets rid of team defense for your leagues. I find this one to be infuriating personally because almost every week there are so many IDPs to pick up that scored more and were on the wire.

'Standard' - 7 total, 2 DL, 2 LB, 2 DB, 1 UTIL (any position)
You can jump to this to start if 3 feels like too few. Having 7 gives you one fewer spot-on defense than offense and means you'll need to do a little pre-season research and know where the tiers are for each position. You will also need to spend FAAB or use waiver wire priority to add an IDP at some point in the season.

Advanced - 7 Total 1 DE, 1 DT, 1 EDGE, 1 LB, 1 CB, 1 S, 1 UTIL
The same total number of IDPs but now we are getting a little more intricate. We need to know how the tiers at each position work and decide if it's worth it to take a DT like Aaron Donald over a higher scoring LB or S because the DT pool is shallow or just risk a low score. It adds a little more strategy for trades and pickups as well.

Expert - 11 Total, 2 DE/EDGE, 1 DT, 2 LB, 2 CB, 2 S, 2 UTIL
1st year in an IDP league and this is the Fantasy Football version of starting on the Black Diamond run as a new skier. This will even make LB a priority as the difference between the 1st and the 40th LB (we'll say half the UTIL are LBs and half Safeties) was about a TD. We are also dealing more with injuries, waivers/FAAB and playing matchups more closely.

I can't convince my league mates to make the switch

Tell them that you guarantee that they will like IDP more than team defense because I haven't met anyone that has tried IDP and preferred team defense after. If that doesn't work maybe try a 2nd free league for a year and see if they prefer it. Also, an IDP only league is very enjoyable, although I prefer having both sides of the ball represented.

My league is a keeper league, how would I add IDPs?

I'm guessing it would come to a league vote but adding a few, maybe 3 to start and 4 the following year and if you all want 4 the next year. You also can do an IDP only draft or auction to add them and then they wouldn't have to be slow rolled. Adding IDPs to your keeper league also makes the NFL draft way more enjoyable, you'll be thinking of fantasy values when guys like Micah Parsons are drafted, he plays ILB and they already have Jaylon Smith and Leighton Vander Esch.

Overall IDP Rankings

1. Darius Leonard, IND (LB1)
2. Devin White, TB (LB2)
3. Bobby Wagner, SEA (LB3)
4. Roquan Smith, CHI (LB4)
5. Blake Martinez, NYG (LB5)
6. Myles Garrett, WAS (DL1)
7. Zach Cunningham, HOU (LB6)
8. Tremaine Edmunds, BUF (LB7)
9. Fred Warner, SF (LB8)
10. Chase Young, WAS (DL2)
11. Jamal Adams, SEA (DB1)
12. Budda Baker, AZ (DB2)
13. Deion Jones, ATL (LB9)
14. Joe Schobert, JAX (LB10)
15. Demario Davis, NO (LB11)
16. Nick Bosa, SF (DL3)
17. Joey Bosa, LAC (DL4)
18. Jeremy Chinn, CAR (DB3)
19. Landon Collins, WAS (DB4)
20. Jessie Bates, CIN (DB5)
21. Aaron Donald, LAR (DL5)
22. DeForest Buckner, IND (DL6)
23. Patrick Queen, BAL (LB12)
24. Jordan Hicks, AZ (LB13)
25. Quinnen Williams, NYJ (DL7)
26. Leonard Williams, NYG (DL8)
27. Jamin Davis, WAS (LB14)
28. John Johnson, LAR (DB6)
29. Jabrill Peppers, NYG (DB7)
30. Jordan Poyer, BUF (DB8)
31. Antoine Winfield, TB (DB9)
32. Jaylon Smith, DAL (LB15)
33. Eric Kendricks, MIN (LB16)
34. Devin Bush, PIT (LB17)
35. Cory Littleton, LVR (LB18)
36. Isaiah Simmons, AZ (LB19)
37. Brian Burns, CAR (DL9)
38. Jason Pierre-Paul, TB (DL10)
39. J.J. Watt, HOU (DL11)
40. Alex Singleton, PHI (LB20)
41. Jamie Collins, DET (LB21)
42. Jerome Baker, MIA (LB22)
43. DeMarcus Lawrence, DAL (DL12)
44. Stephon Tuitt, PIT (DL13)
45. Sam Hubbard, CIN (DL14)
46. Lavonte David, TB (LB23)
47. T.J. Watt, PIT (LB24)
48. Foyesade Oluokon, ATL (LB25)
49. Kenneth Murray, LAC (LB26)
50. Myles Jack, JAX (LB27)
51. Krys Barnes, GB (LB28)
52. Jayon Brown, TEN (LB29)
53. Shaq Thompson, CAR (LB30)
54. Minkah Fitzpatrick, PIT (DB10)
55. Marcus Maye, NYJ (DB11)
56. Logan Ryan, NYG (DB12)
57. Malcolm Jenkins, NO (DB13)
58. Vonn Bell, CIN (DB14)
59. Khari Willis, IND (DB15)
60. Kevin Byard, TEN (DB16)
61. Romeo Okwara, DET (DL15)
62. Cameron Jordan, NO (DL16)
63. Montez Sweat, WAS (DL17)
64. Maxx Crosby, LVR (DL18)
65. Brandon Graham, PHI (DL19)
66. Nick Kwiatkoski, LVR (LB31)
67. A.J. Johnson, DEN (LB32)
68. Eric Wilson, MIN (LB33)
69. Malcolm Butler, AZ (DB17)
70. Marlon Humphrey, BAL (DB18)
71. Trevon Diggs, DAL (DB19)
72. Kareem Jackson, DEN (DB20)
73. Derwin James, LAC (DB21)
74. Justin Simmons, DEN (DB22)
75. Jonathan Abram, LVR (DB23)
76. Dre Greenlaw, SF (LB34)
77. Jordyn Brooks, LAC (LB35)
78. Bobby Okereke, IND (LB36)
79. Dont'a Hightower, NE (LB37)
80. Za'Darius Smith, GB (LB38)
81. Shaquil Barrett, TB (LB39)
82. Anthony Barr, MIN (LB40)
83. C.J. Mosley, NYG (LB41)
84. Micah Parsons, DAL (LB42)
85. Chris Jones, KC (DL20)
86. Cameron Heyward, PIT (DL21)
87. Kenny Clark, GB (DL22)
88. Xavier McKinney, NYG (DB24)
89. Harrison Smith, MIN (DB25)
90. Keanu Neal, DAL (DB26)
91. Justin Reid, HOU (DB27)
92. Tyrann Mathieu, KC (DB28)
93. Fletcher Cox, PHI (DL23)
94. Jonathan Allen, WAS (DL24)
95. Jeffery Simmons, TEN (DL25)
96. Grady Jarrett, ATL (DL26)
97. Akiem Hicks, CHI (DL27)
98. Robert Spillane, PIT (LB43)
99. Jeremiah Owusu-Koramoah, CLE (LB44)
100. Micah Kiser, LAR (LB45)
101. Christian Kirksey, HOU (LB46)
102. Leighton Vander Esch, DAL (LB47)
103. Danny Trevathan, CHI (LB48)
104. Nick Bolton, KC (LB49)
105. Kyzir White, LAC (LB50)
106. Josey Jewell, DEN (LB51)
107. Benardrick McKinney, HOU (LB52)
108. Zaven Collins, AZ (LB53)
109. Chandler Jones, AZ (LB54)
110. Rashaan Evans, TEN (LB55)
111. Troy Reeder, LAR (LB56)
112. Frank Clark, KC (DL28)
113. Trey Hendrickson, CIN (DL29)
114. Emmanuel Ogbah, MIA (DL30)
115. Josh Allen, JAX (DL31)
116. Danielle Hunter, MIN (DL32)
117. Jadeveon Clowney, CLE (DL33)
118. Trey Flowers, DET (DL34)
119. Carl Lawson, NYJ (DL35)
120. A.J. Terrell, ATL (DB36)
121. Kenny Moore, IND (DB37)
122. Richie Grant, ATL (DB38)
123. Trevon Moehrig, LVR (DB39)
124. Adrian Amos, GB (DB40)
125. Arik Armstead, SF (DL36)
126. Derek Barnett, PHI (DL37)
127. Carlos Dunlap, SEA (DL38)
128. Damien Wilson, JAX (LB57)
129. Bud Dupree, PIT (LB58)
130. Von Miller, DEN (LB59)
131. Khalil Mack, CHI (LB60)
132. Harold Landry, TEN (LB61)
133. Haason Reddick, CAR (LB62)
134. Matt Milano, BUF (LB63)
135. Willie Gay, KC (LB64)
136. T.J. Edwards, PHI (LB65)
137. Malik Harrison, LVR (LB66)
138. Clelin Ferrell, LVR (DL39)
139. Shelby Harris, DEN (DL40)
140. Alex Highsmith, PIT (DL41)
141. Chase Winovich, NE (DL42)
142. Yannick Ngakoue, LVR (DL43)
143. Randy Gregory, DAL (DL44)
144. Bradley Chubb, DEN (DL45)
145. Mike Hilton, CIN (DB41)
146. Taron Johnson, BUF (DB42)
147. Marcus Peters, BAL (DB43)
148. Tre'Davious White, BUF (DB44)
149. Anthony Harris, PHI (DB45)
150. Daniel Sorensen, KC (DB46)

DL Rankings

Tier 1

These are the peak Defensive Linemen in the game right now. Garrett has added to his points per game every year he has been in the league. Young averaged over 12 points per game in the last 4 weeks of the season. The Bosa brothers could easily have the 1 and 2 spots here if they didn't have an injury history. Aaron Donald is one of the best Defensive Linemen ever and the only reason Buckner doesn't get more attention in the media.

1. Myles Garrett, CLE (DE)
2. Chase Young, WAS (DE)
3. Nick Bosa, SF (DE)
4. Joey Bosa, LAC (DE)
5. Aaron Donald, LAR (DT)
6. DeForest Buckner, IND (DT)

Tier 2

It shouldn't come as a surprise that the Jets weren't using Leonard Williams correctly because as soon as he traded to the Giants he averaged a career high in points. Quinnen Williams averaged more points than him and was stuck with Gase last year. This year Quinnen gets Robert Saleh and a better offense both should put him in a better position to rush the passer. Brian Burns had a surprising number of tackles and JPP has averaged at least 7.8 points 5 straight seasons. Watt is a bit of a risk in Arizona but with opposing offenses trying to match points he should have a lot of chances at the QB.

7.   Quinnen Williams, NYJ (DT)
8.   Leonard Williams, NYG (DT)
9.   Brian Burns, CAR (DE)
10. Jason Pierre-Paul, TB (DE)
11. J.J. Watt, AZ (DE)

Tier 3

This is the 'consistent with upside' tier of DL to me. Everyone here averaged over 6 points per game last year with the exception of Crosby who played through a torn labrum all year. All defensive lineman and have a bad day but these are some of the least likely to give you nothing,

12. Demarcus Lawrence, DAL (DE)
13. Stephon Tuitt, PIT (DE)
14. Sam Hubbard, CIN (DE)
15. Romeo Okwara, DET (DE)
16. Cameron Jordan, NO (DE)
17. Montez Sweat, WAS (DE)
18. Maxx Crosby, LVR (DE)
19. Brandon Graham, PHI (DE)

Tier 4

This is the same thing as the last tier only for Defensive Tackles. These guys have been consistently making tackles for a while at DT and they all have been able to get to the QB on occasion. Jones offers the most upside and has averaged as much as 8.6 points in 2018. Heyward averaged a high of 9.2 in 2019 but last year's 5.7 was his lowest since 2012. We won't see another DT for a little bit after these guys.

20. Chris Jones, KC (DT)
21. Cameron Heyward (DT)
22. Kenny Clark, GB (DT)

23.   Fletcher Cox, PHI (DT)
24.   Jonathan Allen, WAS (DT)
25.   Jeffery Simmons, TEN (DT)
26.   Grady Jarrett, ATL (DT)
27.   Akiem Hicks, CHI (DT)

Tier 5

This is a 'boom or bust' tier. Not necessarily for their play although guys like Hendickson, Lawson and Clowney will depend on them. This is more about guys that have put up some big seasons in the past getting back to it. That description doesn't really fit Ogbah but he's only had 4 games over 10 points in 3 seasons. Clark didn't have one last year but he had 4 in 2018. Hendrickson and Lawson are moving to new teams. Josh Allen took a huge step back after averaging 6.4 points his rookie year. Flowers, Clowney and Hunter all missed games (Hunter the whole season with a neck injury).

28.   Frank Clark, KC (DE)
29.   Trey Hendrickson, CIN (DE)
30.   Emmanuel Ogbah, MIA (DE)
31.   Josh Allen, JAX (DE)
32.   Danielle Hunter, MIN (DE)
33.   Jadeveon Clowney, CLE (DE)
34.   Trey Flowers, DET (DE)
35.   Carl Lawson, NYJ (DE)

Tier 6

This is the last batch of DL that I actually would trust to roster in a standard 12 man league. Some of them are old vets like Barnett, Dunlap, Suh and Campbell. Others like Ferrell, Highsmith, Winovich, Wilkins and Kinlaw are developing and I'll take a chance and see if this is the year they put it all together but this is the last trustable tier for DL in my opinion.

36.   Arik Armstead, SF (DE)
37.   Derek Barnett, PHI (DE)
38.   Carlos Dunlap, SEA (DE)
39.   Clelin Ferrell, LVR (DE)
40.   Shelby Harris, DEN (DE)
41.   Alex Highsmith, PIT (DE)
42.   Chase Winovich, NE (DE)
43.   Yannick Ngakoue, LVR (DE)
44.   Randy Gregory, DAL (DE)
45.   Bradley Chubb, DEN (DE)
46.   Dre'Mont Jones, DEN (DE)
47.   Christian Wilkins, MIA (DT)
48.   Javon Kinlaw, SF (DT)
49.   Ndamukong Suh, TB (DT)
50.   Calais Campbell, BAL (DT)

Tier 7

The all-upside tier. There is *some* consistency here, guys like Payne, Hughes, Addison and Wolfe. The others are either rookies (Phillips and Paye), young veterans (Lawrence, Payne, Oliver, Gross-Matos), in a new location or starting for the first time.

51.   Jaelan Phillips, MIA (DE)
52.   Kwity Paye, IND (DE)

53.   David Onyemata, NO (DT)
54.   Dexter Lawrence, NYG (DT)
55.   Daron Payne, WAS (DT)
56.   Ed Oliver, BUF (DT)
57.   Jerry Hughes, BUF (DE)
58.   Kerry Hyder, SEA (DE)
59.   Derek Wolfe, BAL (DE)
60.   Mario Addison, BUF (DE)
61.   Shaq Lawson, HOU (DE)
62.   Yetur Gross-Matos, CAR (DE)

The Rest (no particular order)

These are the guys that I would take a flier on an extremely deep league.

Veterans

Robert Quinn, CHI (DE)
William Gholston, TB (DE)
Morgan Fox, CAR (DE)
Dee Ford, SF (DE)
Vinny Curry, NYJ (DE)
Benson Mayowa, SEA (DE)
Dante Fowler, ATL (DE)
Henry Anderson, NE (DE)
Larry Ogunjobi, CIN (DT)
Javon Hargrave, PHI (DT)
Dalvin Tomlinson, MIN (DT)
Malik Jackson, PHI (DT)

Rookies/Young Vets

K'Lavon Chaisson, JAX (DE)
Marcus Davenport, NO (DE)
Josh Sweat, PHI (DE)
Ifeadi Odenigbo, NYG (DE)
Uchenna Nwosu, LAC, (DE)
A.J. Epenesa, BUF (DE)
Joe Tryon, TB (DE)
D.J. Wonnum, MIN (DE)
Charles Omenihu, HOU (DE)
Payton Turner, NO (DE)
Azeez Ojulari, NYG (DE)
Jayson Oweh, BAL (DE)
Derrick Brown, CAR (DT)
Christian Barmore, NE (DT)

Free Agents (I won't rank them until they sign)

Melvin Ingram (DE)
Justin Houston (DE)
Olivier Vernon (DE)
Everson Griffen (DE)
Geno Atkins (DT)
Kawann Short (DT)
Sheldon Richardson (DT)
Jurrell Casey (DT)
Damon Harrison (DT)

LB Rankings

Tier 1

The best of the best among LBs, which means the best of all IDPs. These guys all put up a crazy amount of tackles, stay on the field for all 3 downs and will occasionally put up QB type numbers. Devin White had over 30 points in a game and Blake Martinez and Zach Cunningham had a low of 9 for the whole season.

1.   Darius Leonard, IND
2.   Devin White, TB
3.   Bobby Wagner, SEA
4.   Roquan Smith, CHI
5.   Blake Martinez, NYG
6.   Zach Cunningham, HOU
7.   Tremaine Edmunds, BUF
8.   Fred Warner, SF

Tier 2

These guys all can be in the 1st tier next season and they all had a great 2020. I just have holes to poke with them that I don't with the 1st tier. Jones has been great the past 2 seasons but he was a 1st overall type of player until he had foot surgery in 2018. Joe Schobert played over 1100 snaps last year and with Lawrence in town the defense shouldn't be on the field as much. Davis lacks upside, Queen needs to play better to stay on the field and Hicks has been in trade rumors since the Cards drafted Collins. Once again, all very good LBs and some of the best IDPs but it's easier to see the downside with them than it is tier 1.

9.   Deion Jones, ATL
10.   Joe Schobert, JAX
11.   Demario Davis, NO
12.   Patrick Queen, BAL
13.   Jordan Hicks, AZ

Tier 3
This is where you get your LB2. These guys should all hover around the 10-point mark per game with some big games here and there. TJ Watt will be much higher in leagues that have more points for big plays. The next big play dependent type LB is in tier 5 so Watt is getting a lot of respect here. Davis was a 1st rounder that was brought into stay on the field, I expect him to be more like Queen than Simmons in their rookie years. Simmons is in this tier too after a disappointing 2020 but they have assured us he'll be a starter this year. Kendricks had an amazing 2020 but the Vikings get Barr back so I'm keeping expectations minimal. Devin Bush is coming off an ACL injury but he's the signal caller for Pittsburgh. I might be low on a guy like Collins with the Lions adding some big dudes on the line in front of him. Littleton probably isn't in the same area in skill as these other guys here but the Raiders didn't draft an immediate replacement.

14.   Jamin Davis, WAS
15.   Jaylon Smith, DAL
16.   Eric Kendricks, MIN
17.   Devin Bush, PIT
18.   Cory Littleton, LVR
19.   Isaiah Simmons, AZ
20.   Alex Singleton, PHI
21.   Jamie Collins, DET
22.   Jerome Baker, MIA
23.   Lavonte David, TB
24.   T.J. Watt, PIT

Tier 4
This is a smaller tier that in my opinion just has more guarantees than the next lower tier. Four guys have downsides from their 2020 seasons. Oluokon had by far a career high in snaps, Jack has the same issue as Schobert, Brown had a rough grade (PFF) against the run and that's what keeps LBs on the field and the Panthers added Perryman which should eat into Thompson's production (for the games he's healthy for). Keneneth Murray had a bumpy rookie season and an actual preseason should help him. Krys Barnes is the best inside LB on the Packers roster going into the season and someone has to make tackles there.

25.   Foyesade Oluokun, ATL
26.   Kenneth Murray, LAC
27.   Myles Jack, JAX
28.   Krys Barnes, GB
29.   Jayon Brown, TEN
30.   Shaq Thompson, CAR

Tier 5
This is a tier of high-end 2nd linebackers. Kwiatkowski through Okereke are all guys playing next to the guy expected to make the most tackles. Hightower, Mosley and Barr are all coming off of big injuries. Smith and Barrett

are sack dependent and Parsons is a rookie with 2 big LBs on the roster.

31.	Nick Kwiatkoski, LVR
32.	Alexander Johnson, DEN
33.	Eric Wilson, PHI
34.	Dre Greenlaw, PHI
35.	Jordyn Brooks, SEA
36.	Bobby Okereke, IND
37.	Dont'a Hightower, NE
38.	Za'Darius Smith, GB
39.	Shaq Barrett, TB
40.	Anthony Barr, MIN
41.	C.J. Mosley, NYJ
42.	Micah Parsons, DAL

Tier 6

This is the 50/50 tier; they all have traits that are positives and negatives. Spillane had success for part of a season in Pittsburgh but looked great in his starts. JOK, Bolton and Collins are rookies. Kiser, White and Reeder aren't that good to be blunt. Kirksey, Vander Esch and Jones were all banged up last year. McKinney is playing next to Baker and they'll eat into each other's production. BUT, they all have starting jobs and should be on the field close to 90% of the snaps.

43.	Robert Spillane, PIT
44.	Jeremiah Owusu-Koramoah, CLE
45.	Micah Kiser, LAR
46.	Christian Kirksey, HOU
47.	Leighton Vander Esch, DAL
48.	Danny Trevathan, CHI
49.	Nick Bolton, KC
50.	Kyzir White, LAC
51.	Josey Jewell, DEN
52.	Benardrick McKinney, MIA
53.	Zaven Collins, AZ
54.	Chandler Jones, AZ
55.	Rashaan Evans, TEN
56.	Troy Reeder, LAR

Tier 7

This is a mixed bag. Some here are the biggest names in the NFL because they rush the passer but that leads to huge days and donuts, too much inconsistency (Dupree, Miller, Mack). We also have the no upside LB2s (Wilson, Milano, Edwards), and some first time starters (Gay and Harrison). Reddick has been up and down in his 4 seasons, he's coming off of a career year but also moving teams,

57.	Damien Wilson, JAX
58.	Bud Dupree, TEN
59.	Von Miller, DEN
60.	Khalil Mack, CHI
61.	Harold Landry, TEN
62.	Haason Reddick, CAR
63.	Matt Milano, BUF
64.	Willie Gay, KC
65.	T.J. Edwards, PHI

66. Malik Harrison, BAL

The Rest (no particular order)
These are the guys that I would take a flier on an extremely deep league.

Young and looking for snaps
Pete Werner
Germaine Pratt
Logan Wilson
Akeem Davis-Gaither
Chazz Suratt
Isaiah McDuffie
Baron Browning
Monty Rice
Ernest Jones

Starting LBs that could get replaced
Jon Bostic
Anthony Walker
Nicholas Morrow
Anthony Hitchens
Denzel Perryman
Ja'Whaun Bentley
Kyle Van Noy
AJ Klein
Ty Summers
Malcolm Smith
Sione Takitaki
Jahani Tavai
Reggie Ragland
Neville Hewitt

Rotational pass rushers
Kyler Fackrell
Rashan Gary
Leonard Floyd

Unsigned Free Agents (I won't rank them until they sign)
Kwon Alexander
K.J. Wright
De'Vondre Campbell
Avery Williamson
Tahir Whitehead
B.J. Goodson

DB Rankings

Tier 1
The tippy top, Adams could easily be in a tier of his own but there is upside to everyone here. The Cardinals offense could get even better which would mean more opportunities for Budda. Jeremy Chinn was a rookie last year and should take a step up in his 2nd year. Last year was the first that Collins didn't average over 10 points and that was because of an injury. Jesse Bates is one of the more consistent players I've ever seen, 100 tackles or more and 3 INTs in each of his first 3 seasons.

1. Jamal Adams, SEA (S)
2. Budda Baker, AZ (S)
3. Jeremy Chinn, CAR (S)
4. Landon Collins, WAS (S)
5. Jessie Bates, CIN (S)

Tier 2
A smaller tier, like with the LBs, I trust these guys to be high end DBs a little more than the next tier. John Johnson and Antoine Winfield offer upside too, Johnson is moving to a team that should have late leads which should give him more opportunities. Winfield, like Chinn, was a rookie last year and is on a Bucs team that will still be a throw first team.

6. John Johnson, CLE (S)
7. Jabrill Peppers, NYG (S)
8. Jordan Poyer, BUF (S)
9. Antoine Winfield, TB (S)

Tier 3

These guys have just a little more swing and miss in them. Fitzpatrick is a little big play dependent. Logan Ryan will play S and CB which can lead to some up and down weeks. Maye had his highest scoring season in 2018 (9.7) followed by his lowest scoring season in 2019 (6.1). I'm not sure what to expect from the offense in New Orleans and if it takes a step back that's fewer chances for Jenkins. Bell and Byard have been inconsistent over their careers but should be between 8-10 PPG. Byard I just want to perform at this level two year in a row.

10.   Minkah Fitzpatrick, PIT (S)
11.   Marcus Maye, NYJ (S)
12.   Logan Ryan, NYG (S)
13.   Malcolm Jenkins, NO (S)
14.   Vonn Bell, CIN (S)
15.   Khari Willis, IND (S)
16.   Kevin Byrad, TEN (S)

Tier 4

Big tier here. We first have 2 CBs in Butler and Humphrey that play on teams with high powered offenses. They will get points because they will get thrown at even as good coverage corners. Diggs just wasn't very good last year so he was thrown at, he should get better but so will the Cowboys offense with Dak back. Jackson, Simmons, Abram, Smith, Reid and Mathieu are all solid starters that should average 8-9 points. James has higher end potential as but is injury prone, Neal is the same. McKinney was being used all over the place in his rookie year, he played slot corner and flipped back to safety when Peppers played in the box. He missed the first 11 weeks but will offer versatility this year and should stay on the field for most snaps.

17.   Malcolm Butler, AZ (CB)
18.   Marlon Humphrey, BAL (CB)
19.   Trevon Diggs, DAL (CB)
20.   Kareem Jackson, DEN (CB/S)
21.   Derwin James, LAC (S)
22.   Justin Simmons, DEN (S)
23.   Jonathan Abram, LVR (S)
24.   Xavier McKinney, NYG (S/CB)
25.   Harrison Smith, MIN (S)
26.   Keanu Neal, DAL (S)
27.   Justin Reid, HOU (S)
28.   Tyrann Mathieu, KC (S)

Tier 5

We move down to another hefty tier. We have some corners that get thrown at and make tackles in A.J. Terrell, Hilton and Johnson. Terrell lines up on the outside while Hilton and Johnson are slot corners, they all stay on the field though. We have some rookie safeties that should earn playing time quickly in Grant, Moehrig and Holland. Then more good CBs that get tackles because their opponents are playing catchup with Moore, Peters and White. Amos, Harris and Sorensen are steady vets

29.   A.J. Terrell, ATL (CB)
30.   Kenny Moore, IND (CB)
31.   Richie Grant, ATL (S)
32.   Trevon Moehrig, LVR (S)
33.   Adrian Amos, GB (S)
34.   Mike Hilton, CIN (CB)
35.   Taron Johnson, BUF (CB)
36.   Marcus Peters, BAL (CB)

37.   Tre'Davious White, BUF (CB)
38.   Jevon Holland, MIA (S)
39.   Anthony Harris, PHI (S)
40.   Daniel Sorensen, KC (S)

Tier 6

There's some good CBs in this tier but they cover #1 WRs so they will still get tackles. Carlton Davis, James Bradberry, Xavien Howard and Janoris Jenkins are that group. Consistent yet underwhelming, Safeties in Wilson, Clark, Savage, Jackson and Edmunds. Awuzie, Dunbar, Griffin and Austin had tackles because they were not great. Troy Hill is another high-end slot CB.

41.   Donovan Wilson, DAL (S)
42.   Chidobe Awuzie, CIN (S)
43.   Troy Hill, CLE, (CB)
44.   Quinton Dunbar, DET (CB)
45.   Shaquill Griffin, JAX (CB)
46.   Carlton Davis, TB (CB)
47.   James Bradberry, NYG (CB)
48.   Xavien Howard, MIN (CB)
49.   Bless Austin, NYJ (CB)
50.   Janoris Jenkins, TEN (CB)
51.   Chuck Clark, BAL (S)
52.   Darnell Savage, GB (S)
53.   Eddie Jackson, CHI (S/CB)
54.   Terrell Edmunds, PIT (S)

Tier 7

Tracy Walker, Jalen Mills, Jimmie Ward, Rodney McLeod and Quandre Diggs are veterans with very little upside or downside. Davis, Fuller, Rapp, Jenkins and Curl all have some playing time questions but have a higher ceiling than most. Kazee has a great opportunity in Dallas but he's coming off an Achilles tear.

55.   Ashtyn Davis, NYJ (S)
56.   Tracy Walker, DET (S/CB)
57.   Jalen Mill, NE (S/CB)
58.   Jordan Fuller, LAR, (S)
59.   Jimmie Ward, SF (S/CB)
60.   Rodney McLeod, PHI (S)
61.   Eric Murray, HOU, (S)
62.   Taylor Rapp, LAR (S)
63.   Quandre Diggs, SEA (S)
64.   Damontae Kazee, DAL (S)
65.   Rayshawn Jenkins, JAX (S)
66.   Kamren Curl, WAS (S)

The Rest (no particular order)
These are the guys that I would take a flier on an extremely deep league.

Safeties
Jordan Whitehead, TB
Jarrod Wilson, JAX
Chauncey Gardner-Johnson, NO
Marcus Williams, NO
Nasir Adderley, LAC
Duron Harmon, ATL
Devin McCourty, NE
Amani Hooker, TEN
Tashaun Gipson, CHI
Ronnie Harrison, CLE
Micah Hyde, BUF
Karl Joseph, LVR
Kyle Dugger, NE
Juston Burris, CAR

Corners
Cameron Sutton, PIT
Marshon Lattimore, NO
Jeff Okudah, DET
Jason Verrett, SF
Bryce Callahan, DEN
Cameron Dantzler, MIN
Trayvon Mullen, LVR
Jamel Dean, TB
Jonathan Jones, NE
Joe Haden, PIT
J.C. Jackson, NE
Anthony Brown, DAL
Patrick Peterson, MIN
Jaire Alexander, GB
C.J. Henderson, JAX
Caleb Farley, TEN
Trae Waynes, CIN

Adoree' Jackson, NYG
Sean Murphy-Bunting, TB

Free Agents (I won't rank them until they sign)
Richard Sherman (CB)
Steven Nelson (CB)
D.J. Hayden (CB)
Josh Norman (CB)
Buster Skrine (CB)
Bashaud Breeland (CB)
Gareon Conley (CB)
Kenny Vaccaro (S)
Bradley McDougald (S)
Malik Hooker (S)
Jeff Heath (S)

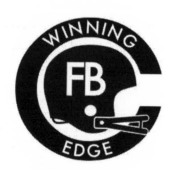

Chapter 11

Dynasty, Rookies & UDFA

Scott Bogman

DYNASTY FIRST YEAR PLAYER PPR MOCK

TEAM	ROUND 1	ROUND 2	ROUND 3
1	Najee Harris, RB - PIT	Pat Freiermuth, TE - PIT	Dyami Brown, WR - WAS
2	Ja'Marr Chase, WR - CIN	Chuba Hubbard, RB - CAR	Amari Rodgers, WR - GB
3	Kyle Pitts, TE - ATL	Rhamondre Stevenson, RB - NE	Tutu Atwell, WR - LAR
4	Travis Etienne, RB - JAX	D'Wayne Eskridge, WR - SEA	Amon-Ra St.Brown, WR - DET
5	Devonta Smith, WR - PHI	Mac Jones, QB - NE	Josh Palmer, WR - LAC
6	Javonte Williams, RB - DEN	Rondale Moore, WR - AZ	Nico Collins, WR - HOU
7	Trevor Lawrence, QB - JAX	Elijah Moore, WR - NYJ	Hunter Long, TE - MIA
8	Jaylen Waddle, WR - MIA	Kenneth Gainwell, RB - PHI	Kyle Trask, QB - TB
9	Trey Lance, QB - SF	Kadarius Toney, WR - NYG	Kellen Mond, QB - MIN
10	Justin Fields, QB - CHI	Trey Sermon, RB - SF	Anthony Schwartz, WR - CLE
11	Terrace Marshall, WR - CAR	Michael Carter, RB - NYJ	Tommy Tremble, RB - NYJ
12	Zack Wilson, QB - NYJ	Rashod Bateman, WR - BAL	Elijah Mitchell, RB - SF

DYNASTY FIRST YEAR PLAYER SUPERFLEX MOCK

TEAM	ROUND 1	ROUND 2	ROUND 3
1	Trevor Lawrence, QB - JAX	D'Wayne Eskridge, WR - SEA	Dyami Brown, WR - WAS
2	Trey Lance, QB - SF	Rhamondre Stevenson, RB - NE	Amari Rodgers, WR - GB
3	Justin Fields, QB - CHI	Rondale Moore, WR - AZ	Pat Freiermuth, TE - PIT
4	Zack Wilson, QB - NYJ	Kenneth Gainwell, RB - PHI	Amon-Ra St.Brown, WR - DET
5	Najee Harris, RB - PIT	Elijah Moore, WR - NYJ	Davis Mills, QB - HOU
6	Ja'Marr Chase, WR - CIN	Kadarius Toney, WR - NYG	Chuba Hubbard, RB - CAR
7	Kyle Pitts, TE - ATL	Kellen Mond, QB - MIN	Tutu Atwell, WR - LAR
8	Mac Jones, QB - NE	Trey Sermon, RB - SF	Josh Palmer, WR - LAC
9	Travis Etienne, RB - JAX	Kyle Trask, QB - TB	Nico Collins, WR - HOU
10	Devonta Smith, WR - PHI	Michael Carter, RB - NYJ	Anthony Schwartz, WR - CLE
11	Javonte Williams, RB - DEN	Rashod Bateman, WR - BAL	Ian Book, QB - NO
12	Jaylen Waddle, WR - MIA	Terrace Marshall, WR - CAR	Hunter Long, TE - MIA

QUARTERBACKS

Trevor Lawrence, JAX (Clemson - Round 1, Pick 1): Trevor Lawrence is the best QB prospect we have seen since Andrew Luck. The first article I read about him had the quote, 'If Peyton Manning could run.' That is, of course, a Steve Nebraska-Esque fantasy, but Lawrence has everything you would want or need to see. He's 6'5" with a giant arm. He didn't lose a single regular-season game in college, won a national title in his 1st season with Clemson, and won all kinds of awards. Lawrence has been the #1 pick in this draft; the wait has been to see who gets it, and Jacksonville didn't screw it up!

- **2021 Value:** It's going to be very high. He goes to an offense that had a little success with Gardner Minshew, and he has weapons in DJ Chark, Marvin Jones, Laviska Shenault, Travis Etienne, and James Robinson. The defense is rough still, so they should be playing catchup in a lot of games. He should push QB1 status this year.
- **Dynasty Value:** Everything you would expect of a player of his caliber, my only fear is if Urban Meyer crashes and burns quickly, they could be playing musical chairs HC or OC. Even if that happens, Lawrence should still be able to be a great NFL and fantasy asset for a long time.

Zach Wilson, NYJ (BYU - Round 1, Pick 2): Wilson put together an unbelievable 2020 season at BYU. He was on the radar before 2020 but not as the 2nd pick behind Lawrence. The most impressive thing to me about him is how he manipulates the pocket and his accuracy downfield. A lot has been made of the lack of top-end competition BYU faced, but it's not like Wilson had a ton of high drafted skill position players like Lawrence, Fields, and Jones. I'm not worried so much about the pressure as I am the potential for injuries. He had shoulder and thumb surgery in 2019 but didn't show any signs of it bothering him in 2029.

- **2021 Value:** He already has better weapons than Sam Darnold ever had in New York, with FA signee Corey Davis, Jamison Crowder, Denzel Mims, and 2nd round pick Elijah Moore coming in. The running game should be in focus under new HC Robert Saleh and OC Mike LaFleur, so he'll be a QB2 in deeper leagues and probably a WW add in standard 12 man leagues.
- **Dynasty Value:** He'll be my QB2 in this class. He may not have the upside in the running game that Fields, Lawrence, and Lance do, but he did have ten rushing TDs in 2020, and he scrambles well. Wilson isn't going to get the benefit of the doubt in New York, the pressure is on, and he's going to need to impress this year not to be rushed out of town, but I think he can do it.

Trey Lance, SF (NDSU - Round 1, Pick 3): The 9ers knew who they wanted, and there may not be a QB in this class with more upside than Lance. The 2020 FCS season was postponed after one game, so he didn't get to play much last year, but he had a 28/0 TD/INT ratio in 2019 and ran for 1100 and 14 TDs. Not playing in 2020 worries some people, but he showed enough in 2019, and the fact he's dripping with potential makes him worth a grab and stash in any dynasty league.

- **2021 Value:** Luckily, he gets to sit and knock the rust off while learning a new playbook and adjusting to the speed of the NFL. Teams don't typically let a QB drafted this high sit for too long, though, so I would expect to see him sooner rather than later, and San Francisco has all kinds of targets for him in Kittle, Deebo, and Aiyuk,
- **Dynasty Value:** He put up video game numbers in 2019 but playing at the FCS level and only one game in 2020 makes him a bit riskier than the other QBs in this class. I talked to Tim Jenkins (Jenkins Elite QB School) in the offseason, and he said NDSU had a bigger talent discrepancy than Alabama. The talent is there for Lance, but his jump from the FCS to the NFL is more prominent than anyone else in this class, an enormous ceiling with a bottom out floor.

Justin Fields, CHI (Ohio State - Round 1, Pick 11): I've been watching Justin Fields since he was on the Netflix show QB1, and he is electric! He's the best athlete in this class of athletic QBs, and he has the attitude and tenacity of a team leader who is a big need for the Bears. Fields had a 67/9 TD/INT, and he can take off and run when he wants (4.46 40 yard dash), although he didn't need to with all the weapons he had at Ohio State. The most impressive thing to me was him playing through broken ribs against Clemson and Alabama in the playoffs. The big knock against him was processing and getting to those 2nd and 3rd reads, but he's going to have great weapons and time to learn in Chicago.

- **2021 Value:** With all due respect to Andy Dalton, I can't imagine that he will keep Fields on the bench. HC Matt Nagy and GM Ryan Pace are on the hottest of seats, so if Dalton doesn't look crisp to start the season, Fields could be in sooner rather than later. The running upside will give him a boost, and he has some great weapons. Probably a great waiver wire add.
- **Dynasty Value:** I have a ton of confidence in Fields himself, and I wouldn't hesitate to draft him. I do worry about the Bears HC/GM situation. If they don't have much success this year, they'll clean house, and the new coaching staff and front office might not like Fields or may want to bring in someone they like. Some QBs never reach their full potential because of bad coaching, or they are rushed to play before they are ready (i.e., Josh Rosen, Mitch Trubisky, Sam Darnold).

Mac Jones, NE (Alabama - Round 1, Pick 15): I love this landing spot for Mac Jones. He can sit behind Cam Newton for most of (if not the entire) season and learn. Even though he's probably the most' Pro ready' outside of Lawrence sitting behind a veteran, learning doesn't hurt QB prospects. The knocks on Mac aren't really about him; he was surrounded by four 1st round WRs, he had the best OL in the country. The real knocks on him are that he doesn't have a cannon arm and doesn't scramble well. He had a 41/4 TD/INT for the most prolific offense in CFB history. He won every award that isn't the Heisman in 2020 (Davey O'Brien Award, Johnny Unitas Golden Arm Award, Manning Award, and Consensus All-American). Josh McDaniels has a pretty good history of working with unathletic QBs that don't have a cannon for an arm; Mac Jones will have every opportunity to succeed in New England.

- **2021 Value:** I think Cam Newton will start for at least ¾ of the season unless he gets hurt, but if Mac does step in, the Pats will most likely run the ball and play conservative, so I don't expect Mac to have a ton of value this year.
- **Dynasty Value:** Mac Jones should take over next season at the latest, and I think he has a ton of potential. I would rank him 5th in this class, but I have him as a solid mid-tier QB2 in dynasty, somewhere between Matt Ryan and Kirk Cousins.

Kyle Trask, TB (Florida - Round 2, Pick 64): Trask is a bit of a mixed bag. The thing I like the most about him is that he improved every year. He went from a redshirt backup to unseating Felipe Franks (a three-year starter) his junior year to being 4th on the Heisman ballot his senior year. He had a 43/8 TD/INT last year and led Florida to the SEC Championship. Tampa Bay has all kinds of talent on the roster at the skill positions, and Trask is a guy that soaks up info football like a sponge. This seems like a perfect fit for his long-term value.

- **2021 Value:** If he's starting games, something is very wrong with Tom Brady, or they are so far ahead he's resting before the playoffs.
- **Dynasty Value:** He's way behind the 1st round guys, but this is the best-case scenario for him. He has sat in the past and waited for his opportunity and made the most of it, and I expect him to do the same in Tampa Bay. There's no one better to learn from than the greatest QB of all time. The only worry is that Tom Brady might play until he's 90 years old.

Kellen Mond, MIN (Texas A&M - Round 3, Pick 66): I didn't give this pick the credit it deserved when it happened. I'm not the biggest fan of Mond (I'm a Longhorns fan and admittedly hate TAMU). However, Mond has the arm talent and can pull it down and run, which has gotten him some comps to Colin Kaepernick, which I think is a bit ambitious. It doesn't matter what I believe, though, as the Vikings are looking to replace Cousins. They tried to trade up for Justin Fields. It's probably more about the $45 mil they have to pay Cousins in 2022 than his performance, but either way, Mond could have a shot at starting in 2022. Mond is a three-year starter with upside, but I'm not interested.

- **2021 Value:** He might not even be the straight backup to Cousins this year; Browning and Stanley are still on the roster.

- **Dynasty Value:** It's more likely that Mond has a chance to start in 2023 when Cousins contract is up, but if they do find a QB desperate team to take him in the offseason, Mond could have a shot at 2022, but he would have to be very impressive in preseason and practices this year.

Davis Mills, HOU (Stanford - Round 3, Pick 67): This pick was weird. The Texans have so many needs and didn't pick until the 3rd round and made Mills their first pick in this draft. Watson might not play this year or ever again, but the Texans have Tyrod Taylor and Ryan Finley on the roster. Mills was a big-time recruit at Stanford but only started part of 2019 and 5 of Stanford's six games in 2020. He has the size at 6'3", 220, and a big arm, but he lacks starting experience and is wildly inconsistent. The tools are there for Mills, but he needs to sit and learn, and the Texans might need a QB soon. I'm not too fond of the fit for him in Houston.
- **2021 Value:** Watson is up in the air, but Tyrod Taylor should start if Watson is suspended or booted from the league. Ryan Finley isn't a great option, but he has starting experience and will probably be the backup to Taylor with Mills being inactive most weeks.
- **Dynasty Value:** The size and arm talent are there, but he needs to sit for a while. I hope for his sake he isn't called upon to start this year.

Ian Book, NO (Notre Dame - Round 4, Pick 133): The bad news is that Ian Book is not a very good QB prospect, in my opinion. He makes some terrible decisions, doesn't have the size or a big arm (it's good but not great), and he doesn't have great touch on his passes. The good news is that he creates with his legs, is a GREAT team leader according to teammates and coaches, and he landed in New Orleans, where they like guys like him (Taysom Hill).
- **2021 Value:** Not much, shouldn't play QB at all but might get some Taysom Hill like work
- **Dynasty Value:** I don't think there's much here, but he couldn't have landed in a better place than New Orleans for his development.

Sam Ehlinger, IND (Texas - Round 6, Pick 218): I LOVED watching Ehlinger play at Texas, and he put up tons of value in CFF leagues. Unfortunately for me, that doesn't mean he's going to be a good NFL player. Ehlinger, to me, is precisely what Tim Tebow was coming into the NFL, a QB built like a LB that runs like a psycho in between the tackles and in the open field. His passing game isn't as great, though, his footwork isn't very crisp, and his arm is below average. I think his peak is as a long-term backup QB who could be in line for some goal-line packages.
- **2021 Value:** Might get a helmet on game days if they decide he's a legit goal-line weapon, but Eason will probably back up Wentz this year.
- **Dynasty Value:** If he evolves to become a starter, he'll put up huge numbers, but I don't think that is a reasonable expectation for him.

RUNNING BACKS

Najee Harris, PIT (Alabama - Round 1, Pick 24): I'm not usually a fan of taking an RB in the 1st, but the need fit for Pittsburgh, and they took the best one on the board. Najee was the Doak Walker award winner and a 1st team All-American for the National Champion Crimson Tide in 2020. He scored 30 TDs while posting 1891 yards and will be the primary workhorse for the Steelers, who were dead last in rushing last year. The comparison to Le'Veon Bell is spot on. He is an incredible runner that can run routes and beat DBs as a receiver from day one. The Steelers line is rough, but he can and will find daylight and bring the running game back to respectable starting week 1.

- **2021 Value:** He's a borderline RB1 in any format but firmly in there for me in a PPR league. He has 530 touches over the last two seasons and carried the load for Bama through the playoffs; he's as proven as they get coming into the NFL.
- **Dynasty Value:** He's going to get the touches on a year-to-year basis. My only concern is how quickly Pittsburgh fixes the OL and who replaces Big Ben at QB. His low-end value is Josh Jacobs, and his high end is peak Le'Veon Bell.

Travis Etienne, JAX (Clemson - Round 1, Pick 25): The best comparison that I've seen made for Etienne is Reggie Bush. Etienne is unbelievably explosive. He averaged 7.8 yards per touch at Clemson and scored 70 TDs over his four seasons. He doesn't need to touch the ball 20+ times to make big plays which is nice because Jacksonville already has a between-the-tackles running back in James Robinson. He's not the purest of pass-catchers, but he improved in that area every year and wound up with 102 in his career, with 85 of those coming over his last two seasons.

- **2021 Value:** I don't buy the Urban Meyer' 3rd down back' stuff we heard when he was drafted. 1st round backs tend not to linger on the bench such that I would expect at least a 50/50 split between Robinson and Etienne. Good RB2, excellent RB3.
- **Dynasty Value:** I love the fact that he landed on the same team with Trevor Lawrence, and he should be able to fit into Urban Meyer's system from day 1. James Robinson is a good back, but he's the type of back that needs touches, he had 289 last season, and there's no way he's going to see that many again. Etienne averaged 18 touches his senior year, and he put up over 7 yards a touch and had 16 TDs.

Javonte Williams, DEN (North Carolina - Round 2, Pick 35): One of the most fun RBs to watch run that I've ever seen. His balance is incredible. He's almost impossible to knock over and has a ton of broken tackles. He's not the most natural at following blocks, but he creates by staying on his feet, and his motor keeps him driving forward every time he touches the ball. The only downside is that we never really had to see him carry the load by himself. He split carries with Michael Carter at UNC and had 20 or more touches only five times.

- **2021 Value:** The Broncos won't have to rely on Williams to carry the load in his rookie year as he'll be behind Melvin Gordon in the pecking order at least to start.
- **Dynasty Value:** He has Aaron Jones-type upside. I would love to see Denver get a QB so opposing defenses don't stack the box, but even with a subpar QB, there are many weapons to account for in Denver, and Williams is a great addition.

Trey Sermon, SF (Ohio State - Round 3, Pick 88): Sermon is an exciting big back to watch, and at the end of the 2020 season, we saw him explode. He put up 331 rushing yards against Northwestern in the Big 10 Championship game and followed up with 31 carries for 192 yards against Clemson in the playoff beat down against Ohio State. Unfortunately, he had some issues with staying healthy, he only had one carry against Alabama, and he dislocated his shoulder. He also had a back injury and knee injury in College. The landing spot is nice in SF because they will ride the hot hand, and Sermon can be streaky. He has way more upside than Mostert and Wilson, and this could be a lovely fit.

- **2021 Value:** The 9ers had two backs go over 100 carries (Wilson 126, Mostert 104), and McKinnon kicked in 81. Shannahan likes to rotate backs, obviously, but Sermon can immediately push for carries, and they will ride the hot hand. A late flyer or WW add for this season.

- **Dynasty Value:** Mostert, Wilson, and Gallman are all UFAs after this season, and I wouldn't be shocked if 2 of them were cut before the season starts. I envision Sermon and Mitchell to be an excellent 1-2 punch in SF.

Michael Carter, NYJ (North Carolina - Round 4, Pick 107): The landing spot is great for Carter. The Jets are looking for some playmaking ability at the RB spot. With Gase gone, we should see a complete offense that can create room for Carter to work in. He's a Phillip Lindsay type in that he's undersized and won't be able to carry the load in the NFL but can still make an impact. He split touches with Javonte Williams at UNC in 2020 and put up 1512 total yards and 11 TDs.
  - **2021 Value:** OC Mike Lafleur will most likely go with multiple backs like San Francisco used; they need to figure out who between Tevin Coleman, La'Mical Perine, Ty Johnson, and Carter will get touches. Luckily Carter can return kicks and punts, so he should get a helmet every week.
  - **Dynasty Value:** Day 3 picks aren't guaranteed anything in the NFL, so he'll have to prove himself, but I like his upside, and he's got an easier path to playing time than most in New York.

Kene Nwangwu, MIN (Iowa State - Round 4, Pick 119): This was one of my least favorite picks in the draft. Nwangwu has tremendous speed (4.31 40 time) and can be explosive in the open field, but his upside as an RB seems pretty limited. He's just not a very instinctual runner, but he is a great special teams player, and that's what I think Minnesota drafted him for, which limits his upside tremendously for fantasy.
  - **2021 Value:** Even if he was drafted to play RB for the Vikings, he's behind Dalvin Cook, Alexander Mattison, and Ameer Abdullah. He should at least be active every week as a special teamer.
  - **Dynasty Value:** I don't want to rule him all the way out because he does have the speed that NFL teams can't teach, and he's a team player, but I don't see it working out for him as more than a change of pace back at his absolute peak.

Rhamondre Stevenson, NE (Oklahoma - Round 4, Pick 120): Stevenson is a big back that can deliver a hit. He always looks smooth running, which is why some had his comp as Arian Foster. However, I think someone like his new teammate Damien Harris is a better comp, personally. Which begs the question, why would the Patriots need a back like they already have? He could quickly push Michel off the roster and have a primary role.
  - **2021 Value:** If he beats out Michel, I expect him to back up Harris for this season. At best, he would lead this team like Harris did last year with somewhere in the neighborhood of 150 carries.
  - **Dynasty Value:** His upside is pretty high, but with the way the Patriots use running backs recently, he could end up a cog in the wheel. He's a complete back compared to LeGarrette Blount, and Blount parlayed that role into 300 touches.

Chuba Hubbard, CAR (Oklahoma State - Round 4, Pick 126): Chuba lost a lot of steam from 2019 to 2020 after suffering an ankle sprain. He never looked the same. He had 328 carries for 2094 yards and 21 TDS for Oklahoma State in 2019. That was cut down to 133 carries for 625 yards over only seven games in 2020, and his YPC went from 6.4 to 4.7. Hubbard obviously has tremendous upside, but he relies too much on his speed, and when he didn't have it at full strength last year, he suffered.
  - **2021 Value:** While backing up CMC has meant standing on the sideline for most of the past. It should mean a little more after he was held to 3 games last season. Even with an uptick, he's more of a handcuff in deeper leagues.
  - **Dynasty Value:** If you own CMC, you should try to find a way to grab Hubbard. Unfortunately for Chuba, McCaffrey is signed through 2025. Hubbard can put it all together, but it's going to take a trade or injury for him to get consistent carries.

Kenny Gainwell, PHI (Memphis - Round 5, Pick 150): I was astonished that Gainwell lasted this long, but he is on the short side at 5'8", but he's rocked up at 200 lbs. It probably had more to do with him opting out, but whatever the reason, the Eagles got a deal. Gainwell offers versatility, playing in the backfield and lining up at WR (51-610-3). He is dangerous with the ball in his hands regardless of how he gets it; he had over 2000 yards from scrimmage in

2019 with 16 TDs. He won't be getting 20 touches a game as he did in Memphis, but he should find a role quickly after making a few big plays.

- **2021 Value:** I feel like Kenny Gainwell is the 2nd best back on the Eagles before even taking a snap. The downside for him is that he slipped to the 5th round, and he didn't play special teams, and he's not a great pass blocker.
- **Dynasty Value:** He has to make a good first impression, but he's my 6th ranked RB in this class, and I think he's the perfect compliment to Miles Sanders.

Elijah Mitchell, SF (Louisiana - Round 6, Pick 194): One of my favorites in this class, legit speed (4.33 40), and he is reliable as a pass-catcher. He was part of a three-headed committee at Louisiana, so he only had 20 touches in 6 games of 42 he played in. He returns kicks, which will help Hilton make the team but with Mostert and Sermon locked in as the #1 and 2 backs, that leaves two spots between Jeff Wilson, Wayne Gallman, JaMycal Hasty, and Mitchell.

Gary Brightwell, NYG (Arizona - Round 6, Pick 196): This one I don't get. I guess Brightwell has perceived upside, and it wasn't like he was set up for success at Arizona. Barkley is the lead back, Booker is behind him, so Brightwell will have to beat at least one of Elijhaa Penny, Jordan Chunn, and Taquan Mizzell.

Larry Rountree, LAC (Missouri - Round 6, Pick 198): Rountree had 793 touches at Missouri against some formidable SEC defenses, and he was productive every year. I don't know that he's any better than Joshua Kelley or Justin Jackson, but they both are league average at best, and the Chargers need someone to compliment Austin Ekeler. Rountree is an excellent inside runner and ok receiving option.

Chris Evans, CIN (Michigan - Round 6, Pick 202): Chris Evans got lost in the shuffle at Michigan after having to sit out in 2019 due to an academic issue. He was a big-time recruit wasted at Michigan because they want to play 15 RBs a game. However, he should have an easier path than some of the other guys drafted in this area because the Bengals let Giovanni Bernard walk and now only have Trayveon Williams and Samaje Perine behind Joe Mixon.

Demetric Felton, CLE (UCLA - Round 6, Pick): He's a weapon more than an RB or WR. He had 1101 yards rushing with 7 TDs and 958 receiving with 8 TDs at UCLA. I love the pick for the Browns, but I don't know how he gets on the field. Chubb, Hunt, and Johnson are the top 3 backs, and the WRs behind OBJ and Landry are Higgins, DPJ, Schwartz, and Hodge.

Khalil Herbert, CHI (Virginia Tech - Round 6, Pick 217): Another RB I like slipping to the end of the draft. Herbert is one of the better pure runners in this class, but he isn't the best pass catcher. I don't think it matters as the Bears seem to have four good backs. David Montgomery will be the lead back, Damien Williams will be right behind him, and Tarik Cohen is the receiving back. Herbert will have to beat out Ryan Nall and Art Pierce to make the team.

Jake Funk, LAR (Maryland - Round 7, Pick 233): Funk is a great athlete, but this is a Special Teams pick. Funk only touched the ball 158 times over four seasons, mainly because he blew out his left knee twice. However, covering kicks and punts should get him a spot on the team, and passing Xavier Jones or Raymond Calais on the depth chart shouldn't be hard for him.

Gerrid Doaks, MIA (Cincinnati - Round 7, Pick 244): Doaks could be a sneaky option for Miami as he is a complete back with experience, but the Dolphins roster already has 5 RBs behind Gaskin that are the same as him in Malcolm Brown, Lynn Bowden, Salvon Ahmed, Jordan Scarlett, and Patrick Laird. All of those guys were better than Doaks leaving college.

Kylin Hill, GB (Mississippi State - Round 7, Pick 256): I can't ignore the explosiveness from Kylin Hill we can see in his film. He might not be the most refined runner, but he can contribute in the passing game from day 1. He only played in 3 games for Mike Leach before opting out, but he caught 23 passes in those games. He'll have to beat out Patrick Taylor and Dexter Williams to get a spot.

Jermar Jefferson, DET (Oregon State - Round 7, Pick 257): Well, the Lions waived Kerryon, so Jefferson has a spot on the roster seemingly locked up. The problem is behind Swift and Williams. There aren't going to be a lot of opportunities for him without an injury.

Javian Hawkins, ATL (Louisville - UDFA): Undersized but explosive back, nothing behind Mike Davis on the roster, so he should make the team.

Jarrett Patterson, WAS (Buffalo - UDFA): Highly productive back at Buffalo, but he is way undersized at 5'6". He reminds me of a smaller version of Devin Singletary. I wouldn't bet on him to make the team.

WIDE RECEIVERS

Ja'Marr Chase, CIN (LSU - Round 1, Pick 5): We've had two incredible WR classes in a row, and Chase would have been my #1 WR in both of them. He's not a physical freak at just over 6' tall, but he does everything well. He is too strong to press and too quick to give cushion too, he has a great catch radius, and he refuses to go down when he gets the ball. He also gets the benefit of reuniting with Joe Burrow, his QB at LSU. Chase did sit out in 2020, but when he last played with Burrow, he put up a ridiculous 84-1780-20 line, and Burrow won the Heisman.

- **2021 Value:** The Bengals have some great WRs in Higgins and Boyd on their roster, but Chase will come in and immediately be the #1 WR for them. Hopefully, they can keep Burrow on his feet this year,
- **Dynasty Value:** I have Chase as my #8 WR in dynasty and #15 overall. The defense is still rebuilding in Cincy, and they'll have to play point-for-point, but with an explosive offense and the benefit of already having a rapport with his QB, he should produce from day 1.

Jaylen Waddle, MIA (Alabama - Round 1, Pick 6): The Tyreek Hill comparisons are a bit overblown mainly because those expectations are ridiculous to expect from even the best College WR. However, the comparison is in the range of reasonable expectations because Waddle is an absolute freak of an athlete. Waddle isn't going to body up WRs, shed tacklers, or high point balls, but he will torch DBs and make huge explosive plays. He'll also return kicks and punts and is extremely dangerous whenever he gets the ball in his hands.
- **2021 Value:** Waddle, like Chase, also benefits from being reunited with his College QB in Tua Tagovailoa. He could be the #1 WR for the Dolphins, but they do have a player in a similar mold in FA signee Will Fuller, and DeVante Parker should be the leading target still, so Waddle will probably be 3rd or 4th his rookie year.
- **Dynasty Value:** I have him as a firm WR2 with a ton of upside. The high-end possibility is that he turns into a Tyreek Hill type. His floor is pretty low, though. He played alongside three other 1st round talent WRs and didn't face many double teams or coverage stacks. I'm not going to be against him, though, even with the concerns.

Devonta Smith, PHI (Alabama - Round 1, Pick 10): The Heisman winner in 2021 landed in a WR-needy offense which should help him produce from the jump. His 2020 season was historic 117-1656-23, and he torched Ohio State in the National Championship to the tune of 12-215-3. Every team knew the ball was going to him, and they couldn't stop it! I'm unoriginal in the comparison, but skinny Marvin Harrison (who was really thin) is easy to compare. Some will be scared off because of his 170 lb frame, but I don't care about that, to be honest. Maybe he's more likely to go out on a big hit, but it's football. Everybody gets hurt. The upside is too good, and he does all the little things well. To me, he's an easy target leader that will be a thorn in the side of DBs for a long time.
- **2021 Value:** The Eagles need a true #1, Greg Ward led them last year with a line of 53-419-6, and their previous 1000 yard WR was Jeremy Maclin in 2014. Ertz may not even be on the team to start the year, so Smith should have every opportunity to lead this team in receptions and yards.

- **Dynasty Value:** I have him one spot ahead of Waddle in my dynasty rankings, he's going to drop in some rankings because of his small size, and that's understandable, but I'm willing to bank on the talent more than the concern. Hopefully, he can develop with Hurts this year, and they can stick in Philly together for a long time.

Kadarius Toney, NYG (Florida - Round 1, Pick 20): Do yourself a favor and pull up a video of Toney's highlights from his time in Florida. He's an unbelievably explosive, quick-twitch athlete who leaves DBs in the dust (4.37 40). He came into Florida as a QB but flipped to WR, so he only started for the Gators last season. He'll need to refine his route running and other intricacies to be an NFL WR, but he averaged 12.9 yards per touch on 89 plays from scrimmage last year as a very raw WR.

- **2021 Value:** The landing spot is rough. The Giants signed Kenny Golladay in the offseason to go along with Sterling Shepard (signed through 2023) and Darius Slayton (signed through 2022). So Toney will have to beat out some experienced options to get as many snaps as possible. He's a WW add in most leagues for 2021.
- **Dynasty Value:** It might take him a little bit to get going with the sound options in front of him, but his talent is insane, and I'm going to bet on it. He's my WR6 in this class, and I have him as a top 100 dynasty pick.

Rashod Bateman, BAL (Minnesota - Round 1, Pick 27): Love the player but hate the landing spot of Baltimore for him. Bateman can be a #1 option even for Baltimore. He set the Gophers single-season receiving record in 2019 with a 60-1219-11 and helped turn the Gophers into a dynamic offense for once. Bateman isn't going to dust DBs or run over defenders, but he'll get open and make tough grabs consistently, which could make him the best receiving option for Baltimore from day 1.

- **2021 Value:** He's the perfect compliment to Marquise Brown, and he's way better than any other WR not named Sammy Watkins on the roster. He'll be on the field in all 3 WR sets, and Watkins hasn't played an entire season since his rookie year, so I expect Bateman to be a contributor at some point this season.
- **Dynasty Value:** Way more valuable here, even for an offense that is so run-heavy. Bateman should be the possession WR to Brown's explosive playmaking and Andrews being the over-the-middle target. He's my WR5 in this class and a great bench with upside for the future.

Elijah Moore, NYJ (Ole Miss - Round 2, Pick 34): I'm not as big of a fan of Elijah Moore as some are, although that doesn't mean I don't respect his talent. His best asset is getting open and making defenders miss in the open field. My concern is that he lined up almost exclusively in the slot at Ole Miss, and he doesn't have a lot of experience facing press coverage or fighting off DBs to make contested catches. It doesn't mean he can't do those things, just that he's going to need to learn on the job. The Jets are a good landing spot for him as they need some good targets to develop with new QB Zach Wilson. The talent is there for Moore. He broke his former teammate AJ Brown's single-season receptions record at Ole Miss in 2020 with an 86-1193-8.

- **2021 Value:** I would be surprised to see Moore have much value in his rookie season as the Jets have the veteran version of him in Jamison Crowder and two big outside options with Corey Davis and Denzel Mims. I wouldn't rule out the possibility of Crowder getting traded, but it was more likely during the draft than it is now. If Crowder is traded or injured, Moore will see a significant amount of snaps.
- **Dynasty Value:** Crowder will be gone after this year at the latest, so I expect Moore to jump on the scene in 2022. Hopefully, he gets a little more seasoning than expected this season, so he can be a significant contributor in the years to come.

Rondale Moore, AZ (Purdue - Round 2, Pick 48): I love Moore. His Freshman year, he led the country in receptions with 114 for 1258 yards and 12 TDs. He did all of that with some brutal play from the QB position against some of the more formidable defenses in the country. However, since his freshman season, he hasn't looked the same. Moore suffered a hamstring injury early in 2019 and only played seven games the last two seasons. Last season he only played three games and was held to 4 in 2019. He has only had 64 catches across his previous seven games. Some knock Rondale because he didn't see too many targets downfield, and he caught the majority of his passes just beyond the line of scrimmage and did his damage after the catch. I feel this was more due to the QB play, but he will have to prove himself either way. The good news is he'll get plenty of chances for receptions in Arizona.

- **2021 Value:** The Cards throw the ball a ton, but he'll still have an uphill battle to see the field. Hopkins is the #1. They also signed AJ Green in the offseason and still have Christian Kirk on the roster. The Cards also still have Andy Isabella and KeeSean Johnson on the roster, and they have some experience.
- **Dynasty Value:** Way more value in a dynasty format. AJ Green is long in the tooth, and Kirk is up after this season. Moore will need to prove himself, but there isn't a better offensive system for a 2nd WR to have success in than the Air-Raid that Kliff Kingsbury runs. I have him as my 7th WR in this class and just inside the top 100 for dynasty.

D'Wayne Eskridge, SEA (Western Michigan - Round 2, Pick 56): This draft is filled with undersized WRs, and Eskridge is another one. Eskridge had a weird career at WMU. He came in as an RB but flipped to WR his Freshman year in 2016. He was a quick learner and led the team in receiving yards in 2017, but his Senior year, they flipped him to play two ways but mainly focusing on CB. He ended up getting a medical redshirt and coming back and putting up his best numbers, 34-784-8. He is not as rounded as some of the other WRs in this class, but he can start for Seattle, and unlike both Moores, he can line up outside and play the slot.
- **2021 Value:** The Seahawks run the ball more than any other team and already have Metcalf and Lockett, both under long-term contracts. He'll be the 4th option at best behind the 2 WRs and Carson. He will at least return punts and kicks, and he averaged 22.3 yards per touch last year for Western Michigan.
- **Dynasty Value:** As mentioned before, he doesn't need a ton of touches to make an impact which is good because it doesn't look like he'll be higher than the 3rd option in the receiving game for at least two seasons.

Tutu Atwell, LAR (Louisville - Round 2, Pick 57): Another short guy off the board! Atwell is more undersized than even Devonta Smith, who has 4 inches and 15 lbs on him. It will be interesting to see how he gets used in McVay's offense as he is primarily a slot option, but he can also play out of the backfield, and he's an experienced kick returner. The Rams have Woods and Kupp signed through 2025, although they could be cut after 2022 for some much-needed cap savings or traded for the same reason. Even if they get one of them off the team, they still have Van Jefferson through 2023.

- **2021 Value:** Not much for this year with the 3 WRs mentioned before plus DeSean Jackson and Tyler Higbee. He'll be a kick/punt returner and gadget player unless there are copious injuries to the WRs.
- **Dynasty Value:** I have a real fear that Tutu is relegated to being a gadget player for the Rams if they don't move one or both of Woods and Kupp. I have him as my 14th WR in this class.

Terrace Mitchell, CAR (LSU - Round 2, Pick 59): Terrace Marshall fell to the bottom of the 2nd round because of a medical flag that popped up late in the process from a broken fibula he suffered during High School. He ran a 4.4 40 yard dash at 6'2", he's got size and speed, which NFL coaches can't teach, and he can play on the outside or be lined up in the slot. Almost ¼ of his College catches went for TDs (23 of 106). He was the #3 option for LSU during their 2019 Championship run behind Justin Jefferson and Ja'Marr Chase. Last year he played seven games before opting out to concentrate on draft prep (with some rough QB play) and averaged over 100 yards per game for the Tigers with a 48-731-10 line.
- **2021 Value:** I think he's the 2nd best option on the Panthers the day he steps on the field behind Moore, but he's going to have to earn it, Robbie Anderson will be ahead of him, and David Moore is an experienced veteran.
- **Dynasty Value:** He was my #5 option before the draft, and he moved up to #4 after even falling to the bottom of the 2nd round when Toney landed with the Giants. Coaches can't teach size and speed, and he has those, plus he ends up back with his old OC Joe Brady with the Panthers. Who knows what they have in him? I think he lights it up sooner rather than later.

Josh Palmer, LAC (Tennessee - Round 3, Pick 77): I like Palmer, but I was surprised to see him go this high. He's the opposite of most of the guys that went in front of him in that he doesn't have size or speed, but he is a great tactician. Clean routes and excellent handwork will keep him on the field, but he has to put it together. His best season at Tennessee (albeit with terrible QB play) was last year. In 10 games, he had a 33-475-4 line. No prospect is ever completely polished coming out of college, but I'm just not sure there's a ton to add for him.

- **2021 Value:** The Chargers had a kind of rotation at their 3rd WR spot between Guyton and Tyron Johnson. I think Palmer can come in and be the 3rd WR from Week 1 for the Chargers.
- **Dynasty Value:** While I am confident enough he will be the Chargers' 3rd WR quickly, I feel like his ceiling is an NFL 2nd WR which would have him as a decent bench option at his peak.

Dyami Brown, WAS (North Carolina - Round 3, Pick 82): Dyami Brown is one of my favorites in this class. To me, he's the better version of Palmer in that they are both about the same size, but Brown is faster and has been way more productive in his career, putting up a 55-1099-8 line last year. He's also the opposite of some others drafted ahead of him as he is almost exclusively an outside WR. He's another dude with an impressive motor that keeps him on his feet after the first hit and creates big plays down the field.

- **2021 Value:** I love the landing spot in Washington. They need SOMEONE to step up next to Terry McLaurin. They signed Curtis Samuel to play the slot, so he'll need to fight last year's 4th round pick Antonio Gandy-Golden for playing time.
- **Dynasty Value:** This year is the big hurdle for him. In my opinion, should he get playing time by the end of the season, he should be there for whatever new QB they'll draft or sign and be part of the plans moving forward.

Amari Rodgers, GB (Clemson - Round 3, Pick 85): The Packers finally did it and drafted Aaron Rodgers (maybe) a WR!! While he's not a game-changer, he can contribute to the Packers playing in the slot and returning punts. He's undersized at 5'9", but he has some impressive credentials. He tore his ACL during spring practice in 2019 but returned in Week 2, and he climbed a Clemson depth chart littered with four and 5-star prospects.

- **2021 Value:** He may not have a 1st round pedigree that Packers fans wanted, but it shouldn't be hard for him to beat out Lazard, St. Brown, or Funchess.
- **Dynasty Value:** I think he has more NFL value than fantasy value. He could easily be one of the better slot options in the league, but the Packers will always lean on Davante Adams and Aaron Jones 1st, and they will almost have to spend an early-round pick on a receiving weapon soon.

Nico Collins, HOU (Michigan - Round 3, Pick 89): A big-bodied WR that will be a better pro than a college player. This is another weird pick for Houston, WR was a need, but they only had five picks in this draft and spent the 1st one on Davis Mills. Nico is big at 6'4" and very fast for his size (4.45 40), but he isn't the most experienced. Honestly, it was amazing he could have a 37-729-7 line in 2019 (opted out of 2020) with Michigan not throwing the ball often.

- **2021 Value:** Well, we know the QB situation is up in the air, and that's going to have a significant impact on the entire WR corps. This year is an uphill battle anyway with Cooks, Cobb, and Coutee in front of him, but the good news for Collins playing time is that all of them have been known to miss games.
- **Dynasty Value:** The best-case scenario is that Watson comes back, and Collins gets to work with him, but I think that Collins can develop into a solid possession WR at best while his floor is a red-zone target.

Anthony Schwartz, CLE (Auburn - Round 3, Pick 91): The Browns made a great pick here, in my opinion. Schwartz speed might be the best trait of any rookie in this class (4.25 40)! Just get the ball in his hands and watch him bolt past defenders on his way to the endzone. Unfortunately, he needs to clean up the intricacies in his game like route running, playing against press coverage, and timing jump balls. But, if he puts it all together, he'll be incredible.

- **2021 Value:** It's doubtful that he will see the field much this year. The Browns run a lot of 2 TE sets to help with the run game, and even when they do have 3 WRs, Higgins is an experienced vet.

- **Dynasty Value:** I'll admit most guys like this burnout, and that is a tangible outcome, but I love the thought of the upside with his crazy speed. I'll take a swing in a deeper league where I already have some established WRs.

Dez Fitzpatrick, TEN (Louisville - Round 4, Pick 109): This was one of the biggest shocks to me from the NFL draft. Fitzpatrick is a reliable target, but he doesn't have any unbelievable traits. He's average height and weight, fast but not exceptional, has excellent routes but not overly impressive. His best season was his Freshman year, and he didn't seem to improve from it.
- **2021 Value:** He did at least land in a good spot in Tennessee as far as opportunity goes. They only have Josh Reynolds locked in with AJ Brown. After that, it's fellow draft pick Racey McMath, Marcus Johnson, and Chester Rogers to compete with.
- **Dynasty Value:** I'm not going to have any shares of him, but the opportunity is there for him, like I said.

Amon-Ra St. Brown, DET (USC - Round 4, Pick 112): Love this pick for the Lions. While St. Brown didn't have incredible highlights, he was very reliable. He had at least five catches in 18 of his 19 games over the last two years. He excels as a route runner and can make contested catches, making him a reliable target that the Lions desperately need after losing Golladay and Jones this offseason.
- **2021 Value:** Higher than most 4th round picks in their rookie year as the targets in Detroit have taken a massive hit. Tyrell Williams, Breshad Perriman, Quintez Cephus, and Geronimo Allison are all that stand in his way of getting on the field.
- **Dynasty Value:** Higher than most with his path to playing time open this year. I have to imagine the Lions will spend a high pick or free agent money on a WR soon, but he can earn his spot this year and build on it. A lot hinges for him on his 2021 performance.

Jalan Darden, TB (North Texas - Round 4, Pick 129): Darden is a big-play threat, but with the Bucs current depth chart, I would expect him to be a special teamer for now. There might be some opportunity for him next season as AB, Chris Godwin, and Justin Watson are all scheduled to come off the books, but I'm not going to bet on it.

Tylan Wallace, BAL (Oklahoma State - Round 4, Pick 131): I'm not super excited about Wallace landing in Baltimore, and he took the biggest hit in my dynasty rankings because of it. I lowered him from 13 pre-draft to 20 post-draft. He was productive at Oklahoma State, but his knee injury in 2019 seems to have slowed him down. My more significant concern than his play is the Ravens drafting not just Bateman ahead of him but also spending picks on Devin Duvernay and James Proche last year and bringing in Sammy Watkins. It seems to me like they will let them all fight for time and play whoever looks best at practice.

Jacob Harris, LAR (UCF - Round 4, Pick 141): There's some debate about whether Harris is considered a WR or TE, but the Rams tuned in the card at the draft, and it said WR. He's tremendous at 6'5" and has excellent body control, but the Rams drafted him to be a Special Teamer. We already went over the depth chart with Tutu, and Harris has a bigger climb than him.

Ihmir Smith-Marsette, MIN (Iowa - Round 5, Pick 157): This seems like a pick that is more for fit than skill. The Hawkeyes run most of their offense with 2 TEs, and the Vikings do that as well. Smith-Marsette was reliable as a target but had some off-field issues. He'll have a decent chance to make the team, but Thielen and Jefferson are the two main targets, and they run the ball a ton.

Simi Fehoko, DAL (Stanford - Round 5, Pick 179): Fehoko has the stuff you can't teach in size (6'4") and speed (4.43 40), but he is a bit rawer than a lot of the WRs in this class. He only has 61 catches over his two full seasons playing for Stanford, and he didn't do anything special. The Cowboys have Amari Cooper and CeeDee Lamb for the foreseeable future, but Gallup is gone in 2022, so there is hope for some future value.

Cornell Powell, KC (Clemson - Round 5, Pick 181): I like this pick for Powell's potential value. Any WR in the Chiefs offense should get a little boost. Tyreek and Kelce are 1-2, but they've been trying to replace DeMarcus Robinson for a while with guys like Hardman, Pringle; they just signed Tajae Sharpe. Unfortunately, Hardman is the only one whose contract is beyond this season. Powell's best skill set was catching passes downfield, and having the best QB in the league could go a long way for him if he impresses early.

Frank Darby, ATL (ASU - Round 6, Pick 187): This is a late flier pick for the Falcons. He plays faster than his 40 (4.59) time, but he's never really produced, only 67 catches over four seasons with Arizona State. However, Arthur Smith has worked some magic with guys like Firkser and Humphries in Tennessee, so that I won't rule him out.

Marquez Stevenson, BUF (Houston - Round 6, Pick 203): Buffalo is littered with talent at WR. Stevenson was drafted as a kick returner (3 KR TDs the last two seasons) with some upside.

Shi Smith, CAR (South Carolina - Round 6, Pick 204): He was a constant producer at South Carolina, undersized at 5'9", but he's fast and has a high motor. Guys picked in the 6th round and later have to make it on Special Teams. He returned kicks with a 21.3-yard average.

Racey McMath, TEN (LSU - Round 6, Pick 205): He has some size at 6'2 and speed with a 4.39 40, but he only had 33 catches over four seasons at LSU. They drafted him to be a Special Teamer.

Jalen Camp, JAX (Georgia Tech - Round 6, Pick 209): Another Special Teams pick, Camp had 48 catches over four seasons at Tech.

Seth Williams, DEN (Baylor - Round 6, Pick 219): This one legitimately surprised me. A lot of people liked Williams more than his teammate Schwartz. He was a decent producer as well, with 132 catches over three seasons with 17 TDs. He's a big target at 6'3" and can make some contested catches, but the Broncos are deep at WR and TE. He'll have to play some special teams to make the team.
Dazz Newsome, CHI (North Carolina - Round 6, Pick 221): Newsome was a great producer at UNC but falling this far means he's more viewed as a special teamer, he returned kicks during his days at UNC, and that will most likely be his role for Chicago.

Michael Strachan, IND (Charleston - Round 7, Pick 229): This pick isn't a Special Teams pick this late. It's more of a developmental selection. Strachan is a 6'5" track athlete with an enormous two seasons in 18' and 19' at Charleston, 77-2326-27. Hilton will be gone soon, and outside of Pittman, the Colts don't have any other WR spots locked up for the future, so he has a better chance than some guys drafted in this range.

Tre Nixon, NE (UCF - Round 7, Pick 242): Nixon has some speed but doesn't play at his 40 time (4.44). Maybe the Patriots see something they can develop in him.

Ben Skworonek, LAR (Notre Dame - Round 7, Pick 249): Must be another pick for Special Teams. Skowronek was injured in his last two seasons and is another 'tweener' type like Jacob Harris, who they took in the 4th. Longshot to make the team, in my opinion.

Kawaan Baker, NO (South Alabama - Round 7, Pick 256): There is a need for WR in New Orleans as they don't have much behind Michael Thomas, but a 7th round pick three spots from Mr. Irrelevant isn't going to be the answer. Baker can play some special teams, but Deonte Harris and Marquez Callaway have NFL experience and are good enough kick returners. I like Baker, he can play out of the backfield too, but he's guaranteed nothing.

Dax Milne, WAS (BYU - Round 7, Pick 258): Milne was productive with Zach Wilson last year (70-1188-8) and had reliable hands. However, I don't think he has the speed or moves to get open often enough in the NFL.

Cade Johnson, SEA (South Dakota State - UDFA): I was surprised he wasn't drafted, he was an outstanding producer over three seasons at South Dakota State (162-2872-28), and the Seahawks don't have much after Lockett, Metcalf, and Eskridge.

Jonathan Adams, DET (Arkansas State - UDFA)

Sage Surratt, DET (Wake Forest - UDFA): These guys are in the same boat. Adams has a great catch radius but had issues with drops. Surratt has the size, too but is slow. They will be competing against each other for a spot.

TIGHT ENDS

Kyle Pitts, ATL (Florida - Round 1, Pick 4): Rare and generational have been used to describe him, and they are both correct. He's 6'5" with 4.4 flat speed, can body up CBs and burn LBs. He isn't the best blocker, but he's passable and works hard to get better. His best trait for fantasy is getting in the endzone; he scored 12 TDs on 43 catches last season. He can be in the Kelce and peak Gronk range if he reaches his potential.

- **2021 Value:** TEs don't typically do well in their rookie seasons. Fant was pretty good for Denver 50-642-3 in his rookie year. I'm going to have Pitts at four behind Kelce, Kittle, and Waller. He's probably going to be a terrific deal compared to them, so this could be the best year to get him.
- **Dynasty Value:** He has the chance to be in the current day Kelce and peak Gronk. He's my 3rd prospect overall in this class and a top 50 overall prospect.

Pat Freiermuth, PIT (Penn State - Round 2, Pick 55): The 'Baby Gronk' moniker is not even close, but I've heard him compared to fellow Nittany Lion Jesse James, and I don't think that's fair either. He suffered a shoulder injury that held him to 4 games in 2020, but he put more than enough on film in 18 and 19. He's an ok blocker, but he shines in everything we want as fantasy players, route running, getting open, catching the ball, and getting into the endzone.

- **2021 Value:** Pittsburgh isn't the best landing spot for him. They have great receiving options in Juju, Diontae, Claypool, and an accomplished pass-catching TE in Eric Ebron. He'll be a waiver wire add for this year.
- **Dynasty Value:** Ebron can be cut after this year, and Freiermuth could be ahead of him by that point anyway. He doesn't have a Tier 1 TE upside, but his peak could have him in the 2nd Tier if he hits his peak with guys like Fant and Goedert.

Hunter Long, MIA (Boston College - Round 3, Pick 81): I've seen him compared to Austin Hooper, and I think that's a pretty solid one. He led TEs in catches in College Football last year (57-685-5), and he can block playing for Boston College in a run-heavy system.

- **2021 Value:** Probably not a lot as the Dolphins have Gesicki, Shaheen, and Smythe on the roster, who are all built in a similar mold as Long.
- **Dynasty Value:** The good news is that Gesicki and Smythe are UFAs after this season, and he's a way more complete player than Shaheen.

Tommy Tremble, CAR (Notre Dame - Round 3, Pick 83): Another player will be a better pro than a college player. He's already a pro-level blocker, which will benefit the #1 overall pick in Christian McCaffrey, and it will keep him on the field to improve as a pass-catcher. He only had 35 catches and 4 TDs over two seasons, but they didn't need him to be a pass catcher at Notre Dame.

- **2021 Value:** Probably better than expected as he should see the field quickly, Ian Thomas was rough last year, but he's a developing pass catcher that shouldn't be relied on.
- **Dynasty Value:** He's a risky pick as he hasn't displayed much pass-catching prowess, but he's a gamble that's worth taking, in my opinion.

Tre' McKitty, LAC (Georgia - Round 3, Pick 97): This was a surprising pick to me. McKitty was an average blocker with below intermediate receiving skills. However, I'm guessing the Chargers see something here that most didn't, and he can at least sit and learn behind Jared Cook for a season. Cook and Parham are free agents after this year, so he'll have a shot at playing time next season if he shows enough.

John Bates, WAS (Boise State - Round 4, Pick 124): Bates was a surprise to me in the 4th, but Washington does need a little bit more from the position, and Bates can block. Bates doesn't have much upside in the receiving game. His four-year total receiving line was 47-579-2. I don't see much upside for fantasy.

Kylen Granson, IND (SMU - Round 4, Pick 127): I like Granson as a pass-catching option in the NFL. He played as a traditional TE, H-back, and lined up as a WR. His four-year line was 129-1879-16. Indianapolis could be friendly for him too. Eventually, Mo Allie-Cox will be gone, and the receiving options for next year clear out with Hilton becoming a free agent. Nothing is guaranteed, but I like his potential.

Luke Farrell, JAX (Ohio State - Round 5, Pick 145): This seems to me to be Urban Meyer drafting a player he recruited to Ohio State. Farrell's best season was Meyer's last one at Ohio State, so maybe there's something there, but I'm not going to bet on it,

Brevin Jordan, HOU (Miami - Round 5, Pick 147): I'm guessing Jordan dropped because of his injury history at Miami, but he was considered by most to be the 3rd ranked TE going into the draft. He was very productive at Miami. Last year he had a 38-576-7 line. Houston has Jordan Akins on the roster now, but he's a free agent next year, so the plan will be for Jordan to replace him.

Noah Gray, KC (Duke - Round 6, Pick 162): Gray is a natural pass catcher who ran great routes and was a reliable target at Duke; however, he isn't a blocker. The Chiefs drafted him as a TE, so he will most likely stay at that position, but he'll need a lot of work to get a spot on the team, and even if he does, the Chiefs have Kelce.

Zach Davidson, MIN (Central Missouri - Round 6, Pick 168): Weird hybrid punter/TE who didn't even play TE until his Sophomore season at Central Missouri. According to PFF, he was an All-Mid American punter three years in a row, and Colquitt was ranked 32 out of 33 punters. The punting job might earn him a roster spot and allow him to develop as a tight end.

2022 Prospects to Know

QB

Spencer Rattler, Oklahoma (Jr): Big time recruit that is a little undersized but has a big arm and was very impressive as a first year starter in 2020. I don't think his ceiling is as high as Hurts or Murray for fantasy, probably more like Baker.

Kedon Slovis, USC (Jr): Slovis didn't look as sharp in his Sophomore season as he did in his Freshman season but the PAC-12 shutdown and picked back up again late in the process so he'll have a lot riding on his 2021.

Sam Howell, North Carolina (Jr.): Another QB that took a bit of a step back in 2020, it will be interesting to see how he does as a Junior when his 2 leading rushers (Javonte Williams, Michael Carter) and leading WRs (Dyami Brown, Dazz Newsome) were drafted this year.

More to know: Desmond Ridder, (Cincinnati -Sr), Tyler Shough (Texas Tech - Jr), Malik Willis (Liberty - Sr), Phil Jurkovec (Boston College - Jr), JT Daniels (Georgia - Jr)

RB

Isaiah Spiller, Texas A&M (Jr): Spiller is a complete back that has put up some nice numbers for the Aggies, Ainias Smith who plays WR and RB could be drafted next year as well.

Breece Hall, Iowa State (Jr): Enormous season at Iowa State in 2020 279-1572-21, he also can catch 23-180-2.

Mo Ibrahim, Minnesota (Sr): He has averaged over 5 yards per carry 3 years in a row for Minnesota. He'll have to get better in the pass game to move up boards.

More to know: Zamir White (Georgia - Jr), Jerrion Ealy (Ole Miss - Jr), Kevin Harris (South Carolina - Jr), Kennedy Brooks (Oklahoma - Sr)

WR

George Pickens, Georgia (Jr): Big time recruit that has had some rough QB play so far in his career. Has had immaturity issues but the talent is immense.

Chris Olave, Ohio State (Sr): Surprising that he came back when Justin Fields left but the 2021 class was pretty deep at WR and he has a much better chance to go in the 1st round in 2022.

John Metchie, Alabama (Jr): Another potential Bama 1st round WR, we may be getting Bama fatigue but Metchie is a stud.

More to know: Garrett Wilson (Ohio State - Jr), David Bell (Purdue - Jr), Justyn Ross (Clemson - Sr), Treylon Burks (Arkansas - Jr), Jahan Dotson (Penn State - Sr), Khalil Shakir (Boise State - Sr)

TE

Charlie Kolar, Iowa State (Sr): Big time part of the best Iowa State team maybe ever. 7 TDs 2 seasons in a row and a 13.4 career YPC.

Jalen Wydermyer, Texas A&M (Jr): Wydermyer was the Kellen Mond's #1 target for the Aggies last season, Baylor Cupp was the big time recruit but he broke his leg right before the 2019 season and Wydermyer stepped and has proven himself.

More to know: Jeremy Ruckert (Ohio State - Sr), Cade Otton (Washington - Sr), Braden Galloway (Clemson - Jr), Jake Ferguson (Wisconsin - Sr)

Chapter 12

Team Previews

AFC EAST

Kate Magdziuk

Buffalo Bills Fantasy Preview

Key Losses: WR John Brown, G Brian Winters

Key Additions: WR Emmanuel Sanders, QB Mitch Trubisky

The Bills released WR John Brown as a cap casualty back in March to free up $8 million in cap space for the 2021 season. Incredibly, this low-key loss is probably the most significant shakeup for the Bills' offense. Brown has accounted for 167 targets over the past two seasons, averaging 9.1 yards per target. Interestingly, with Brown active, the Bills have averaged 25.08 points per game in their 24 contests and 26.62 points per game without him.

To make up for the loss, the team signed veteran wideout Emmanuel Sanders in his age-34 season. He totaled 7266 receiving yards and five touchdowns in 2020 with the New Orleans Saints, achieving a season-high 122 receiving yards on 14 targets against the Chargers in Week 5. Sanders isn't bound to make a big-time fantasy impact but could be an attractive late-round value in best-ball formats.

NFL Draft Picks of Fantasy Impact: T Spencer Brown, WR Marquez Stevenson
Despite the rumblings that the Bills would be taking a running back in the first round of the 2021 NFL Draft, they left the pick without a single one. Instead, they focused more heavily on defense, taking edge rushers with their first two picks. They did add WR Marquez Stevenson of Houston in the sixth round. However, it's unlikely that we'll see any fantasy-relevant impact given their current WR depth chart.

Offensive Outlook: The Buffalo Bills are, once again, in an excellent spot for the 2021 NFL season — as long as QB Josh Allen is under center. They scored an average of 102.5 fantasy points per game as a unit, ranking fourth among NFL teams. It isn't easy to imagine them doing anything less. Allen officially finished as a top-six fantasy QB in two consecutive seasons and had nine games with 25 or more fantasy points. WR Stefon Diggs will continue to be the de-facto No. 1, and barring injury, has a solid chance to lead the NFL in targets and receiving yards for the second year running.

Alongside Allen will work WRs Cole Beasley (coming off a career-high 82 catches for 967 receiving yards) and second-year wideout Gabriel Davis. Beasley should continue to have sneaky PPR upside after averaging just under 14 fantasy points per game in the 2020 season. We can give thanks to his volume from the slot, having finished each of his seasons with the Bills averaging 7.1 targets per game. TE Dawson Knox remains in the mix as well but isn't an option for fantasy managers. He has yet to exceed 50 targets in a season, averaging just 5.3 fantasy points per game in the 2021 season. Even in a barren tight end landscape, you can indeed find better value elsewhere.

Though the run game (or lack thereof) is less than desirable, the fact that the Bills didn't draft or sign any running back of significance does give RBs Devin Singletary and Zack Moss some value in the coming season. They're likely to continue to split touches pretty evenly, as they did in the final eight games of the 2020 NFL season, where Singletary and Moss saw 80 touches and 77 touches, respectively. For fantasy purposes, it's worth noting that Moss saw 11 attempts inside the five-yard line to Singletary's six — making him the preferred end zone back. However, with Allen's rushing upside, it's hard to trust either of these backs in your lineup in any given week.

Defensive Outlook: Heading into the draft, the team's biggest need was at defensive end, and they addressed it with their first two picks with Gregory Rousseau and Carlos Basham Jr. Outside of edge rushers, they don't have any other glaring holes defensively. Tre'Davius White continues to rank among the league's best cornerbacks, with Tremaine Edmunds up at linebacker and Jordan Poyer at safety — among the league's best. In 2020, Poyer ranked sixth among safeties in total tackles, adding two forced fumbles and two interceptions to his resume to boot. On paper, their defense should continue to be one of the league's better units. However, in 2020, their most significant liability was in the red zone, where they ranked 28th among NFL defenses.

2021 Team Outlook:
Outside of the loss of John Brown, the Bills did a great job of "getting the band back together." They've built a complete roster, top to bottom, offense and defense, and it's difficult to find many deficiencies outside of their run game. The good news is, they've transitioned well into the role of a pass-first team. What more is there to say? The Bills are likely to finish the 2021 season top-five in fantasy points scored once again, with most of them coming from the quarterback and wide receiver position.

New York Jets Fantasy Preview

Key Losses: QB Sam Darnold, RB Frank Gore, WR Breshad Perriman, DE Henry Anderson, LB Tarell Basham

Key Additions: WR Corey Davis, DE Carl Lawson, LB Jarrad Davis, DT Sheldon Rankins

It would appear that the Jets are finally headed in the right direction. This offseason, the organization cleaned house. They hired former 49ers defensive coordinator Robert Saleh to be their head coach. From there, the rebuild began. The team had long been tied to quarterback Zach Wilson, and it seemed that the rumors were all but confirmed when they traded away QB Sam Darnold. They received a 2021 sixth-round pick in addition to a 2022 second and fourth-rounder in compensation, clearing the path for a fresh start at quarterback with rookie Zach Wilson.

NFL Draft Picks of Fantasy Impact: QB Zach Wilson, G Elijah Vera-Tucker, WR Elijah Moore, RB Michael Carter
After drafting BYU QB Zach Wilson with the No. 2 overall pick, the team wasted no time in getting him some help on the offensive line. The Jets traded up from No. 23 to No. 14 to draft OG Alijah Vera-Tucker for protection. Vera-Tucker entered the draft as NFL Draft analyst Daniel Jeremiah's third-highest ranked offensive lineman in this class, deemed one of the "safest players in this draft class."

The team continued to build around Wilson with WR Elijah Moore and RB Michael Carter in the second and fourth rounds, respectively. Though Moore is on the smaller size at 5'9" and 178 pounds, he finished the 2020 NCAA season ranking second in receiving yards and a stunning contested catch rate of 73%, playing most of his snaps from the slot. Carter is also undersized at 5'9 ½" and 184 pounds — ranking in the 12th and 17th percentiles among running backs, respectively. He's well-rounded with back-to-back seasons of 1,000 or more rushers and a more than capable receiver out of the backfield.

Offensive Outlook: Despite the team's shiny new quarterback, there are still plenty of reasons to be cautious when evaluating the Jets' offense in the 2021 NFL season. Let's start with a reminder of what the offense accomplished in 2020. They ranked dead last among NFL offenses in scoring, third-down conversion, yards per play, 31st in big-play rate, passing offense, and PFF grade in pass protection. Simply put, the Jets were a mess, and there's plenty of uncertainty as to how much progress this roster will make in a single offseason.

As far as the passing game goes, Wilson has a strong arm, excellent mobility in the pocket, and his ability to throw off-platform is reminiscent of Patrick Mahomes. However, the Jets receiving corps still leaves something to be desired to offer their rookie quarterback a true alpha WR1. There's indeed plenty of potential there with the likes of 2020 second-round pick Denzel Mims and 2021 second-round pick Elijah Moore, but target distribution and player development remain questions. Free-agent acquisition Corey Davis is coming off a career season with the Titans, where he totaled 984 receiving yards and finished as the WR31 in half-PPR scoring formats. Though he may naturally fill the team's WR1 role, he has yet to exceed 1,000 receiving yards or 5 TDs in a single season. Considering the downgrade, he's facing in the offense, he continues to project as a WR3 with upside.

The rest of the depth chart looks pretty barren, including the depth charts at running back and tight end. Rookie RB Michael Carter will compete with Lamical Perine and Tevin Coleman for touches, neither of which exceeded 3.6 yards per rush attempt in the 2020 season. Chris Herndon remains the team's lead tight end, who did show promise after an impressive 2018 rookie campaign. He totaled 502 receiving yards and 4 TDs, but since, he's averaged just two receptions per contest.

Defensive Outlook: Outside of their rushing defense, which allowed just 4.0 yards per rush attempt (sixth-lowest among NFL teams), the Jets unit was largely just below average in 2020. The few signings they made in free agency for DE Carl Lawson, DT Sheldon Rankins, and LB Jarrad Davis aren't likely to move the needle significantly. Likewise, their secondary is still expected a bottom-10 unit. Look to Quinnen Williams to continue to make an impact as a run defender and pass rusher, but otherwise, the Jets won't be a daunting matchup for opposing offenses.

2021 Team Outlook:
It's difficult to shake the sense of dread in an organization recovering, but the New York Jets seem to be taking the appropriate steps to rebuild their organization. That being said, this is still a team that is still very much in rebuild mode, and their value in dynasty leagues is more significant than their value in redraft.

New England Patriots Fantasy Preview

Key Losses: G Joe Thuney, S Patrick Chung, CB Jason McCourty

Key Additions: WR Nelson Agholor, WR Kendrick Bourne, TE Jonnu Smith, TE Hunter Henry, LB Matt Judon

After signing QB Cam Newton to a one-year extension, the New England Patriots were aggressive in 2021 NFL free agency. They made moves to acquire the top-two available tight ends on the market in Jonnu Smith and Hunter Henry. However, they were less aggressive in terms of pursuing available wideouts. Their top WR signing came in Nelson Agholor, who is coming off a career-high 896 receiving yards.

NFL Draft Picks of Fantasy Impact: QB Mac Jones, RB Rhamondre Stevenson
The New England Patriots had been tied to quarterback Mac Jones throughout the pre-draft process, but I'm not sure anyone would have projected he'd fall right into their lap at No. 15. Due to his lack of mobility and precision as a passer, there's been plenty of comparisons of Jones to another very successful quarterback in Patriots history — Tom Brady. Jones has been highly praised for his football IQ, but his overall lack of rushing upside lowers his ceiling in fantasy football leagues considerably. RB Rhamondre Stevenson just further crowds the running backs room.

Offensive Outlook: Though New England did add the two best tight ends available in 2021 free agency, they still do have a lot of work to do in terms of getting back to the Patriots of yesteryear. Bill Belichick has stated that Cam Newton is set to be the team's quarterback heading into this season, and if that's the case, he should be considered a low-end QB1 with weekly upside due to his rushing ability. He finished his first season with the Patriots totaling 595 rushing yards and 12 TDs, but he failed to achieve as a passer for all he accomplished with his legs. He averaged just 177 pass yards per game (43rd-fewest) and just eight total passing touchdowns to pair with ten interceptions. Newton has admitted that there were times that he did struggle with the playbook, particularly after spending crucial time away from the team after being diagnosed with COVID-19 in Week 4. Another year in the system, we should hope to see Newton's touchdown rate increase from the 2.2% we saw in 2020 closer to his career average of 4.4%, which would have him as a fringe QB1, assuming he starts the entire season. Should Jones earn the starting role at some point, he's unlikely to be of significant value outside of two-quarterback or Superflex format leagues given his lack of rushing upside.

The running backs and wide receivers' rooms are just as perplexing as ever following the 2021 NFL Draft and free agency period. First, RB Sony Michel is a no-go for fantasy managers after scoring fewer than seven fantasy points in five of his nine games played in 2020. Then comes RB Damien Harris, who had a mini-breakout in his sophomore season. He led the running backs in rush attempts and yards per game but saw seven total targets in his 251 offensive snaps. Last but not least, we have veteran James White. If there's any hope for fantasy production among this running back group, it's with him — in PPR formats, at least. White had a down season but continues to be heavily involved as a receiver. He hasn't seen fewer than 62 targets in a single season since 2015 and is the de-facto third-down back, particularly with the departure of RB Rex Burkhead in free agency.

In terms of receiving weapons, the team did get a slight upgrade in WR Nelson Agholor this offseason. After earning a full-time role with the Raiders in Week 3 of 2020, Agholor went on a 16-game pace for nearly just under 1,000 receiving yards and 8 TDs. He joined WRs Jakobi Meyers and failed experiment N'Keal Harry. Enter: the tight end room. After running 12-man personnel groupings just 22 times in the 2020 season, the team went all out to get a jumbo package in TEs Jonnu Smith and Hunter Henry. Though the crowded tight end depth chart has some fantasy managers shying away from drafting either, they are certainly worth consideration considering the continued lack of quality receiving options at wideout.

Defensive Outlook: The Patriots defense had one of its more disappointing seasons in the Bill Belichick-era, but they did have some opt-outs on the defensive side of the ball that should be set for a 2021 return. Additionally, after a one-year stint in Miami, LB Kyle Van Noy returned to Foxborough. Additionally, they signed DE Yannick Ngakoue and LB Matt Judon from the Ravens, who combined for 81 total pressures, including 13 sacks, 43 tackles, and four forced fumbles. These moves put them closer to the margin of a good-to-average defense.

2021 Team Outlook:
The 2021 NFL season seems like it will be one of tradition for the Patriots. Fantasy football managers will continue to play "Guess Who?" at each skill position for who's set for a week of production (and guess incorrectly most times thanks to the mind of Bill Belichick). There are fantasy points to be scored in this offense, mainly if Newton can take the next step forward in learning the playbook. However, the best values in this scheme are likely to be the ones where you don't need to set a lineup. The Patriots continue to win the "best team to draft for best-ball" award annually.

Miami Dolphins Fantasy Preview

Key Losses: QB Ryan Fitzpatrick, LB Kyle Van Noy, DT Davon Godchaux

Key Additions: WR Will Fuller, CB Jason McCourty, C Matt Skura

You could argue that the Miami Dolphins said more with their lack of moves in the offseason than they did with their acquisition. The team let backup RB Ryan Fitzpatrick walk in free agency and traded the No. 3 overall pick in the 2021 NFL Draft to the San Francisco 49ers. With that pick, they could have had a crack at one of the consensus top-end quarterbacks. Instead, they elected to move out of that spot and grab QB Tua Tagovailoa, a receiving weapon. They also signed WR Will Fuller to a one-year deal, thought of as one of the best available receivers in this free agency class. Fuller is suspended for the first game of the NFL season, but when he's on the field and healthy, he provides speed and explosiveness to the offense.

NFL Draft Picks of Fantasy Impact: WR Jaylen Waddle, T Liam Eichenberg

The Dolphins also brought Alabama WR Jaylen Waddle into the mix with the No. 6 overall pick in the draft to reunite with his former Alabama teammate. Though they have experience playing together, his splits with Tagovailoa under center versus QB Mac Jones are worth noting. In the 2019 season, Waddle played nine games with Tagovailoa, totaling 315 receiving yards and two touchdowns. Unfortunately, Tagovailoa then suffered his season-ending hip injury. Waddle then played out the rest of his career with Jones. In eight total games with Jones spanning the 2019 and 2020 NCAA seasons, Waddle totaled 795 receiving yards and 8 TDs. In the second round, they added offensive tackle Liam Eichenberg out of Notre Dame. In 951 pass-blocking snaps in the last two seasons, Eichenberg didn't allow a single sack. He's an instant upgrade at left tackle.

Offensive Outlook: QB Tua Tagovailoa had a disappointing rookie season but has plenty to be optimistic about heading into 2021. With Ryan Fitzpatrick out of town and another year removed from a traumatic hip injury suffered in his final season with Alabama, Tagovailoa may just be feeling a bit more comfortable this season. Among quarterbacks that played at least 25% of snaps in 2020, Tagovailoa ranked 26th among quarterbacks in fantasy points per dropback (two spots ahead of fellow rookie QB Joe Burrow) and 28th in adjusted completion percentage. However, the addition of receivers like Jaylen Waddle, who he played with at Alabama, and Will Fuller are massive upgrades for Tua. They could help him take the next step as a developing quarterback. Because the hype train was so strong heading into his rookie season, Tagovailoa is set to be a late-round value at the QB position in 2021 fantasy leagues.

At running back, the Dolphins are set to employ 2019 seventh-round pick Myles Gaskin as their leading rusher. Though he lacked efficiency with just 4.1 yards per attempt in his second season, starting in Week 3, he assumed a workhorse role that Gaskin maintained through the end of the season. Gaskin played from Week 3 onward in the eight games he averaged just under 16 rush attempts and 4.5 targets per game. Volume is king in fantasy football, and he's likely to be one of the last running backs off of the board that has legitimate potential for 275+ touches in the 2021 season.

As for the receiving corps, the Dolphins have done an excellent job of surrounding Tagovailoa with talented wide receivers. Will Fuller ended his 2020 campaign prematurely after being issued a suspension for PEDs, but in his 11 games played, he was averaging 80 receiving yards and 0.7 touchdowns per game. He was dominating as a true WR1 while on the field, ranking as the WR5 in half-PPR formats. Also worth noting, "TE," aka slot receiver Mike Gesicki takes a hit in value after these wide receiver additions, based on a likely decrease in target volume.

Defensive Outlook: Under Brian Flores, the Dolphins defense has "Flor-ished." Their unit finished the 2020 season leading the NFL in turnovers, allowing the sixth-fewest points and 10th in total sacks. In addition, cornerback Xavien Howard earned First-Team All-Pro honors in his 2020 season after recording ten interceptions, ten pass breakups, and a passer rating of 53.4 when targeted — the second-lowest among any DB to play more than 25 snaps on the season. The addition of Jason McCourty is a big plus too. The Dolphins D/ST finished fourth in fantasy points scored in the 2020 season, and they should continue to be a dominant unit moving forward.

2021 Team Outlook:

In his second year as an NFL head coach, Brian Flores brought the Dolphins to a 10-6 record and got dangerously close to earning a bid to the 2020 NFL playoffs. Barring any complications, they should look to make a run in the 2021 postseason. The offense has enough weapons to take a step forward in their efficiency.

AFC NORTH

Kate Magdziuk

Pittsburgh Steelers Fantasy Preview

Key Losses: RB James Conner, Maurkice Pouncey, TE Vance McDonald, LG Matt Feiler, CB Steven Nelson, LB Bud Dupree

Key Additions: None

Despite the number of players that the Steelers lost in free agency, there hasn't been much of a shakeup with the skill players on offense outside of an upgrade at running back via the NFL Draft. Ben Roethlisberger returns to the team another year removed from a season-ending elbow injury, and WR JuJu Smith-Schuster signed a one-year extension to remain with the Steelers through 2021.

NFL Draft Picks of Fantasy Impact: RB Najee Harris, TE Pat Freiermuth, G Kendrick Green
Following the departure of RB James Conner, the Steelers made no effort to keep their infatuation with Alabama's lead back a secret. They drafted Najee Harris at the No. 24 overall pick, who is set for an instant three-down role in the offense. In the 11 games that starting RB James Conner played at least 50% of offensive snaps, he averaged just under 16 touches per game. Give that to Harris, and he's a lock for a top-15 season, regardless of the offensive line. TE Pat Freiremuth of Penn State also joins the skill position players in Pittsburgh — a luxury pick in the second round, but arguably the second-best tight end in the class behind only Kyle Pitts. Freimuth is a talented receiver with the strength to make an impact as an inline blocker immediately. Considering the team's current WR corps, it doesn't seem likely that Freiermuth is set for a prominent role as a receiver early on in his career. However, he could be pretty valuable when provided the target share.

Perhaps one of the more underrated players with enormous impact potential is interior offensive lineman Kendrick Green. Green comes to the NFL with versatility, playing snaps effectively at both the left guard and center positions over the last two seasons. PFF ranked him as the seventh most highly graded run blocker among the offensive linemen in the 2021 draft class.

Offensive Outlook: The Steelers offensive line is likely to be the team's biggest issue heading into the 2021 season, and they didn't do much to address it in free agency or the 2021 NFL Draft. They lost Maurkice Pouncey in retirement and Alejandro Villanueva to the Ravens in free agency. Still, they will look forward to welcoming back right tackle Zach Banner, who will return from a torn ACL suffered in Week 1 of the 2020 season. There is reason to remain hopeful for Banner, though, who beat out their 2018 third-round draft selection, Chukwuma Okorafor, for the starting right tackle job.

Outside of the offensive line, there's not much to question when it comes to the offense. Among quarterbacks with at least 300 dropbacks in the 2020 season, Ben Roethlisberger had the fifth-shortest average depth of target at 7.4 yards and still managed a QB14 finish in fantasy football leagues; thanks in part to the massive passing volume. He's thrown at least 32 passing touchdowns in each season since 2016, excluding his brief 2019 campaign. So in single-quarterback leagues, he's a viable late-round target on volume and upside alone.

Every quarterback needs a receiving corps, and you'd be hard-pressed to find a trio of three wideouts with higher upside anywhere outside of the 'Burgh. Yet, somehow, Diontae Johnson continues to be significantly undervalued in PPR formats after ranking fifth among NFL wideouts with 144 targets in the 2020 season. He finished the season as fantasy's overall WR22 on the year, but in games where he played more than 25% of offensive snaps, he averaged 17.5 fantasy points per contest. He did register 15 drops on the season, but it's worth noting that 14 of them came after suffering a concussion in Week 3. Concussion symptoms can vary widely among, but Johnson can expect challenges in spatial awareness.

Though Johnson has been the favorite for targets since being drafted, WRs JuJu Smith Schuster and Chase Claypool still managed to make a splash as the WRs 18 and 19 in half-PPR formats, respectively. Each of these wideouts saw at least 110 targets, 930+ receiving yards, and 10+ touchdowns in the 2020 season. Though they ranked back to back in fantasy points, Smith-Schuster did out touch Claypool with 110 receptions, ranking fourth among NFL wideouts on the season. Claypool saw a higher average depth of target and had a higher touchdown rate. Deciding between the two in 2021 fantasy football leagues is likely to come down to your league's scoring format. In PPR scoring formats, Smith-Schuster gets the edge. In non-PPR scoring formats, Claypool's the guy. Either has an opportunity to be a value in 2021 leagues, though, each seeing an average draft position around WR30 as of May.

Last but not least is TE Eric Ebron. Ebron ranked fifth among tight ends in targets and receptions and 11th in receiving yards in his first season with the Steelers. He's finished as a top-15 tight end in five of his last six NFL seasons and had just three games where he scored fewer than five fantasy points in 2020. I'm loving the potential for Ebron's draft position to continue to fall leading up to the 2021 season, particularly as folks fear the prospect of Pat Freiermuth. In redraft leagues, I'm not concerned. Did somebody say "late-round value"?

Defensive Outlook: Though the Steelers defense crumbled slightly towards the end of 2021, it was primarily due to some extensive injuries. T.J. Watt put together a solid campaign to earn defensive player of the year in 2020, tying Rams defender Aaron Donald with 15 sacks and making 23 tackles for loss. In addition, five batted passes, two forced fumbles, and an interception to boot. He and safety Minkah Fitzpatrick each earned first-team All-Pro honors in the 2020 season for their dominant performances.

Despite losing playmakers Bud Dupree and Devin Bush, their 2020 unit tied for second-fewest net yards per pass attempt allowed in the NFL (5.3), fifth-fewest touchdowns allowed (22) tied for a league-high 18 interceptions. They'll return healthier in the 2021 season, which will be critical considering some of the depth lost in the secondary.

2021 Team Outlook:
Despite the narrative surrounding the Steelers' offensive line, they have all of the necessary skill players to continue to be a productive offense. The Steelers have ranked top-four in fantasy points scored by the wide receiver position in each of Roethlisberger's last three full seasons as a starter, and it's unlikely to change now as they make their final push towards a Super Bowl run. The addition of Najee Harris makes me all but certain this team will be one of the most productive teams for fantasy football in the NFL in the 2021 season.

Cleveland Browns Fantasy Preview

Key Losses: None

Key Additions: S John Johnson, CB Troy Hill, DE/OLB Jadaveon Clowney, LB Anthony Walker

The Cleveland Browns didn't see a significant shakeup in personnel this offseason, making their offense a bit easier to project for fantasy football managers. Instead, they made some critical defensive signings in free agency and resigned WR Rashard Higgins to a one-year extension.

NFL Draft Picks of Fantasy Impact: CB Greg Newsome II, Jeremiah Owusu-Koramoah, WR Anthony Schwartz
This was more of a defensive draft for the Browns and a successful one at that. The team drafted cornerback Greg Newsome II out of Northwestern at No. 26 and paired him with LB Jeremiah Owusu-Koramoah of Notre Dame in the second. Owusu-Koramoah was ranked as Daniel Jeremiah's 15th best player available in the draft (even ahead

of Newsome). Still, his draft stock fell after rumored concerns regarding a possible heart condition arose at the NFL's medical combine.

In the third round, the team drafted WR Anthony Schwartz of Auburn — one of the fastest wide receivers in this draft class... or any draft class. Schwartz posted a 4.26 40-yard dash, ranking in the 99th percentile among wideouts, and ranked seventh among NCAA wideouts in yards after the catch in 2020 despite ranking 24th in total targets. Schwartz may not be set to see enough volume to be fantasy relevant on any kind of a regular basis, but his top-end speed will always leave him with a high ceiling and potential for big games.

Offensive Outlook: As it turns out, a Kevin Stefanski-led offense is a pretty significant upgrade to Freddie Kitchens. QB Baker Mayfield took a big step back in his sophomore season under Kitchens, registering a 59% completion rate and near-1-to-1 touchdown-to-interception ratio, but he bounced back big-time in 2020. Mayfield finished the season with a career-high 4,030 passing yards, 165 rushing yards, and a 95.7 passer rating. That being said, he wasn't particularly relevant for fantasy football. In his three years in the NFL, he has yet to rank higher than QB20 in fantasy points per game finishes, and that's likely to continue moving forward. As long as Stefanski is leading the regime, Mayfield ranks as a mid-to-high-end QB2.

There to take pressure off of the passing game is one of the best running back duos in the NFL — Nick Chubb and Kareem Hunt. Both finished as top-10 running backs in the 2020 season, combining for just under 400 total fantasy points on the season. In both Stefanski's seasons as offensive play-caller, his teams have finished top-six in rush attempts, rushing yards, and rushing touchdowns. They're set for much of the same in 2021. Hunt is likely to emerge as the better value in 2021 fantasy leagues, given his lower ADP compared to Nick Chubb's first-to-second round value in fantasy drafts.

At wide receiver, Odell Beckham Jr. is set to return from a torn ACL suffered in Week 7 of the 2020 season. Despite his former status as a top-five dynasty wide receiver, his production has suffered since joining the Browns. WR Jarvis Landry also finished with career lows in targets, receptions and tied for a career-low 4 TDs. These wideouts are competing with tight ends David Njoku and Austin Hooper for targets, too. With a low-volume passing offense and quarterback who likes to spread the ball around, the fantasy football production for these receiving weapons is likely to continue to suffer.

Defensive Outlook: The Browns have a legitimate shot to be one of the league's best defenses in 2021. No, I'm not kidding. Myles Garrett is locked and loaded for another dominant season, registering 56 total pressures and a career-high 32 tackles, and four forced fumbles in the 2020 season. Also, returning is defensive tackle Sheldon Richardson and cornerbacks Denzel Ward and Greedy Williams, who have struggled with staying healthy early on in their careers. Outside of the two defensive rookies we've already noted, the team added safety John Johnson and cornerback Troy Hill, previously with the Rams, and Jadeveon Clowney is joining from the Titans. This crew is set to take 2020's middle-of-the-pack defense into a top-tier unit in the seasons to come. Watch out, AFC North.

2021 Team Outlook: I'm not sure that there's been a single season in recent memory that has favored the browns so highly before it kicks off. Take a look at the offense: 2018's No. 1 overall pick — QB Baker Mayfield — with any combination of RBs Nick Chubb and Kareem Hunt with WRs Odell Beckham Jr., Jarvis Landry, Rashard Higgins, and TEs Austin Hooper and David Njoku? It's a lethal combination to opposing defenses and probably for your fantasy football teams, too, if you're hoping for mass production outside of the running backs room. The Browns ranked 28th in pass attempts and 24th in passing yards in 2020, and with the pack this team is punching defensively, we should continue to expect a run-heavy scheme where they look to control the clock.

Baltimore Ravens Fantasy Preview

Key Losses: RB Mark Ingram, OT Orlando Brown, DE Yannick Ngakoue, LB Matt Judon

Key Additions: G Kevin Zeitler, OT Alejandro Villanueva, WR Sammy Watkins

The Baltimore Ravens lost several key players in the 2021 offseason on both sides of the ball. Mark Ingram left the team in free agency to sign with the Houston Texans, leaving 2020 second-round back JK Dobbins and Gus Edwards to carry the load. Edwards was set to become a restricted free agent in the 2021 season, and the Ravens applied a second-round tender to keep him a year longer. In addition, there were several shifts on the offensive line, including the acquisition of former Giant Kevin Zeitler and former Steeler Alejandro Villanueva. Finally, ahead of the draft, the Ravens traded two-time Pro Bowl tackle Orlando Brown to the Kansas City Chiefs in exchange for several picks, including a 2021 first-round pick.

NFL Draft Picks of Fantasy Impact: WR Rashod Bateman, WR Tylan Wallace, G Ben Cleveland
With the No. 27 overall first pick, the Ravens drafted Minnesota WR Rashod Bateman, who entered this draft as one of this class's more complete receivers with stats and tape to appease analytics and film buffs alike. He recorded a breakout age of 18.8 in his sophomore season (93rd percentile among wideouts), commanding a 35.7% target share (98th) and achieving a 40% dominator rating (81st). His 2020 season wasn't ideal, but his route-running ability speaks for itself. The team went on to draft G Ben Cleveland in the third round as part of their offensive line rebuild, followed by WR Tylan Wallace in the fourth round — another wideout set to appeal to the analytics crowd with his advanced metrics, including a 42.3% dominator rating, 31.3% target share and a breakout age of 19.3.

Offensive Outlook: After finishing as 2019's QB1 in fantasy football with a 9% touchdown rate, Lamar Jackson came back down to earth. He finished as the QB9 in fantasy points per game after seeing a decrease in pass attempts, completion percentage, and touchdown rate, with a bump in his interception rate. Additionally, Jackson stands as the only quarterback in NFL history to rush for 1,000 yards in two straight seasons. His rushing ability gives him the ultimate upside with the maximum floor. However, unless we see some increased volume or efficiency as a passer, we may not see him continue to hold perennial top-five value as a dynasty quarterback.

The Ravens have finished first in the league in rush attempts in each of the last three seasons and first in rushing yards for the past two. The Ravens have a very clearly established identity, and that's unlikely to change significantly regardless of how much desire OC Greg Roman may have to stimulate the passing attack. JK Dobbins finished as the RB24 in his rookie season as the ultimate picture of efficiency. He finished with 6.0 yards per carry — first among all running backs — while ranking 48th in touches per game. Gus Edwards will continue to see kist around 140 touches, as he has done for three consecutive seasons.

The passing scheme in Baltimore is tight end friendly with a 27.8% target share — the fifth-highest rate in the NFL. However, given the low passing volume, that's not saying much for the fantasy potential of the wide receivers. Marquise Brown finished the 2020 season ranking as the WR34 in half-PPR formats as the team's lead wide receiver and a 24% target share. Adding Sammy Watkins, Rashod Bateman, and Tylan Wallace into the mix is likely to be the straw that breaks the camel's back in terms of any single wideout achieving sustainable fantasy value.

Defensive Outlook: In the 2020 season, the Ravens defense allowed the 7th fewest yards per play, second-fewest points, and forced the 10th most turnovers. However, it's possible that with the losses of Yannick Ngakoue and Matt Judon, this unit sees some regression. Ngakoue and Judon combined for 81 total pressures, including 13 sacks, 43 tackles, and four forced fumbles, and their offense may need to help compensate for those losses.

2021 Team Outlook:

The biggest shakeup for the Ravens came at the offensive line and via defensive losses, though they did make some moves in the draft and free agency to fill the gaps. A decrease in defensive efficiency could force them into more passing situations. Still, overall, they'll continue to be a run-first unit with massive fantasy upside across the board as long as it's outside of the wide receivers' room.

Cincinnati Bengals Fantasy Preview

Key Losses: CB William Jackson, DE Carl Lawson, RB Giovanni Bernard

Key Additions: DE Trey Hendrickson, CB Mike Hilton

The most notable off-season loss for fantasy football managers is that of back up running back Gio Bernard. Bernard has been a team-favorite for third-down work and targets to the running back position, leaving the opportunity wide open for touches in the coming season. QB Joe Burrow has also continued on in his rehabilitation process after a season-ending ACL injury and is seemingly on pace for a timely 2021 return.

NFL Draft Picks of Fantasy Impact: WR Ja'Marr Chase

Many made the case that the Bengals should have made a move to draft offensive line with the No. 5 overall pick. Not Joe Burrow, though. It was no secret heading into the 2021 NFL Draft that 2020's No. 1 overall pick was hopeful that the team would draft former LSU teammate, WR Ja'Marr Chase. Chase was the consensus WR1 in the pre-draft process despite opting out of the 2020 season due to COVID-19. In the 2019 season, Chase led the NCAA with 1,780 receiving yards and 20 touchdowns. He ranked top-five in passer rating when targeted, ranked fifth among wideouts missed tackles forced and maintained a 50% contested catch rate — all with LSU teammate Justin Jefferson leading the team with 111 in receptions. Chase was an integral part of LSU's championship win in the 2019 season, and his previous chemistry with Burrow under center is without question.

Offensive Outlook: The Cincinnati Bengals offense is fresh and loaded with talent and ready to score some fantasy points in the 2021 season. In his rookie season, QB Joe Burrow was on pace to attempt 646 passes while completing 65% of passes and a 3.2% touchdown rate. Neither the defense nor the offensive have improved significantly enough to assume increased efficiency in the rushing game or relieve a continuous need to "play catch up" and rack up garbage time yards and points. Burrow ranked 17th in fantasy points per game in his rookie season but also managed an average of 269 pass yards per game. Though Burrow's ceiling as a rushing quarterback may be a bit lower as he returns from injury, his ceiling in dynasty remains quite high with the artillery of weapons the team has placed around him.

RB Joe Mixon is a likely lock for a top-10 finish, particularly with the release of Giovanni Bernard. Mixon saw 23.3 touches per outing in the 2020 season, averaging 16.6 fantasy points per game — ranking 10th best among running backs. He saw a career-high 4.3 targets per game. Since Mixon was drafted in 2017, Bernard has seen an average of 52.5 targets per season, and it seems that as long as Mixon is healthy, he is set to see them.

There are no tight ends worth noting in Cincinnati for fantasy football managers. The depth chart is thin as floss. Starting TE Drew Sample finished the year as the TE39 in 2020 over 16 games. The real meat in this offense is at wide receiver, a corps rich with two dominant outside wide receivers in Tee Higgins and Ja'Marr Chase with Tyler Boyd lining up in the slot.

The general consensus in the fantasy football community has been to fade the Bengals receiving corps. However, considering the potential for passing volume and the quality of the weapons on the field, it's possible that we, as a group, are miscalculating. Though Ja'Marr Chase is extremely likely to see an immediate target share considering his relationship with Burrow, it's definitely worth taking a look back to the 2020 season. In Weeks 1-11 with Burrow under center as the starter, WRs Tyler Boyd, Tee Higgins and AJ Green all saw between 70 to 86 targets. With Joe Burrow, each of these starting wideouts saw between 7 and 9 targets in the end zone. Given the even dispersal share and lack of reasoning to project a decreased passing volume, I'm inclined to believe that Burrow will distribute the ball just as evenly in his second season under center. If any of them sniffs a 20% target share, they're nearly bound for a top-24 finish in this offense, as long as the core of it remains healthy.

Defensive Outlook: The team's defensive losses in Carl Lawson and William Jackson feel like tit-for-tat exchange for Trey Hendrickson and Mike Hilton. If anything, these moves left them with a downgrade. There's been no notable improvement defensively that should have us believing we'll see a more balanced unit heading into the 2021 season. A top-10 passing offense (at least in volume if not in efficiency) should be expected in order to keep up with any defensive deficiencies.

2021 Team Outlook: On paper, the Cincinnati Bengals are looking like every fantasy managers dream. Pair their less-than-ideal defense with a young and talented quarterback, set to reunite with the wideout that helped lead to his championship season in 2019, with a running back that should easily touch the ball 300 times? It's a dream. If Joe Burrow enters the 2021 NFL season healthy, we could very well be in for a top-15 scoring offense in fantasy football leagues, specifically at the wide receiver position.

AFC SOUTH

Chris McConnell

Tennessee Titans Fantasy Preview

Key losses: Malcolm Butler (CB), Adoree` Jackson (CB), Adam Humphries (WR), Jonnu Smith (TE)
Nearly all the critical losses for the Titans this offseason were on defense, but for a good reason (more on that later). First, Butler was brought into Tennessee in 2018 on a five-year deal but never lived up to expectations. The cut cleared $10M in the cap for the Titans. Next, the team earned another $10M in available funds by letting go of Adoree Jackson, who at one time was probably one of the best young corners in the game, but couldn't overcome continuous injuries. Finally, Adam Humphries departs to Washington, leaving a hole at the slot receiver position. The Titans failed to address this early in the draft, so it could be up to someone like rookie Dez Fitzpatrick to fill that void.

Key additions: Bud Dupree (OLB), Janoris Jenkins (CB)
The release of Butler and Jackson allowed the Titans enough cap to send a 5-year, $82.5M deal towards Bud Dupree. Dupree comes in after tearing his ACL in December but is expected to be ready to rock before the season kicks off. Bud is also expected to improve the Titans pass rush from 2020 that ranked 31st in pressure rate (17.6%) and 30th in sacks (19). Janoris will be 33 when the season starts but is still a rock-solid player in the secondary and should help tighten Tennessee's pass defense in some capacity.

Drafted Players of Fantasy Note: Caleb Farley (CB)
The biggest name to know from the Titans draft was arguably the best CB in the class pre-injury. Farley fell further than he usually would have due to injury concerns, but the Titans may have found their next lock-down corner if healthy. They hope he's the answer as their problem in a tough AFC is stopping their opponents from scoring. Farley has a chance to be the best year-on CB draft pick in your IDP league rookie drafts.

Fantasy Impact:
The Titans added a tackle in round 2 of the draft in Dillon Radunz. This should continue to help this O-line properly block in front of Derrick Henry, the star of the Titans' show, and who should return in 2021 as a top 5 fantasy RB. He's a workhorse, he stays healthy, and they feed him the rock like crazy. What's not to like? It remains to be seen how former OC Arthur Smith's departure to Atlanta will affect the offense and Derrick Henry specifically, if at all.

Everyone loves A.J. Brown as the Titans undisputed alpha WR1. AJB finished 2021 as WR14 in PPR leagues. With Adam Humphries and Jonnu Smith departing, Brown may have an even larger target share than he did in 2020, and the sky seems to be the limit as long as Ryan Tannehill continues his solid play under center. Don't hesitate to swipe up AJB in as many fantasy drafts as you possibly can. He's a high-end WR2 at worst. Speaking of filling voids, Anthony Firkser will step in for Jonnu Smith at TE and has the looks of a sneaky pick super late in drafts as a possible TE1 candidate as the team's primary pass-catching TE.

Offensive outlook:

Former OC Arthur Smith leaves for the head job in Atlanta and is generally credited with getting the most out of Tannehill, Henry, and the offensive line. However, the same system is expected to stay in place, so not much should change. This means you can confidently take Derrick as an RB1 yet again in drafts and should be able to capture A.J. Brown as your WR1/2 on your team as well. Both Brown and Henry shouldn't be doubted, but this offense will hum only as good as Ryan Tannehill allows it to. If we get more QB2 consistent production from Tannehill, this offense shouldn't skip a beat in 2021. As mentioned before, Anthony Firkser should be on your radar later in drafts if you're looking for a TE that should provide some low TE1 production. It may be difficult to repeat as the NFL's 3rd overall offense, so some regression should be expected but not enough to alarm anyone hoping for continued production.

Defensive outlook:

This will be the unit that determines more than anything where the Titans wind up at season's end. The only NFL defenses that were worse than the Titans? The Lions, Falcons, Texans, and Jaguars. That tells you just how bad they needed Bud Dupree & Janoris Jenkins in free agency. Those two alone should help the Titans improve on last year's putrid performance, but they will need their young defensive talent to step up if they want to flip this unit into one of the NFL's Top 15 for 2021.

2021 Outlook:

With the Texans and the Jaguars in this very winnable division, the Titans should only have trouble with a Colts team that will likely sport an elite defense and even better offense with Wentz under center. Even then, with the added playoff spots, the Titans can still find their way into the playoffs even if they don't win the division. The favorites to win the crown will likely be the Colts, but it's not like the Titans haven't thrived off being doubted and underappreciated for the last several years, so they probably have all the doubters right where they want them. I don't expect the offensive unit to have much trouble giving the league fits, but as mentioned before, the defense will determine the success of this team. But having Derrick Henry put the team on his back may make that job a bit easier than one would generally imagine.

Indianapolis Colts Fantasy Preview

Key losses: No key losses of note

Key additions: Carson Wentz (QB)

Colts got their QB. Carson got his weapons and his O-Line and his running game, and his coaching/play-caller. What I'm getting at is that Carson has no excuses anymore. He has everything he needs to be once again one of the best players in the NFL and a finalist for league MVP. Too often, we saw Carson put the Eagles on his back and will them to victory or competitiveness. Last year, not so much. But as we know, it wasn't all his fault. I believe his new scenery and a new arsenal of weapons puts Wentz back on the map as a full-fledged QB1 in fantasy and makes the Colts an even more dangerous Super Bowl contender in the AFC.

Drafted Players of Fantasy Note:

There are no drafted players on offense that will make a 2021 impact. For IDP leagues, Kwity Paye is an excellent selection. Widely thought of as the best DE in the draft, he should pay immediate dividends for the Colts and improve their already top ten defense.

Fantasy Impact:
Carson Wentz is the bus driver now, and as he goes, the Colts will go. This was a massive get for Indy as they needed an athletic QB with escapability to get away from defenders; Something Rivers couldn't do last year. Wentz immediately upgrades the outlook of Pittman, Hilton, Taylor, and the rest of the crew as long as they can protect him. Behind arguably the best OL in football, that shouldn't be an issue, and we should see Michael Pittman have a solid sophomore campaign while T.Y. Hilton shows more consistency week to week. Jonathan Taylor, already entering the season as an RB1, has his arrow pointing up as much as ever. JT should have no issues besting his rookie season across the board (health permitting) and has a real shot at finishing as the overall QB1.

Offensive outlook:
The Colts exited 2020 with the 14th ranked offense in the league. That can, and should, definitely be improved upon in 2021, barring injuries. There's nothing this offense doesn't have. It's going to be a lot of fun to watch the Colts this season, and we should fully be expecting Carson and Taylor to be in Tier 1 of their positions this season. Don't be afraid to pair them up in drafts. Hilton should improve on last year's numbers, but it still won't be enough to approach what we came to expect from him back during the Luck era. Michael Pittman is a guy that should be on every single dynasty team you have. He'll take over as the alpha receiver this season and should leave a heavy mark in fantasy circles. He's got 'breakout" written all over him.

Defensive outlook:
This top 8 defense from 2020 only improves after having 3 of their first four picks come on the defensive side of the ball. One of those is Kwity Paye. Probably the best DE in the draft, Paye should be a day one impact player for Indy and help create a terrifying duo alongside DeForest Buckner. As always, though, this defense starts and ends with Darius Leonard. I fully expect the Colts to repeat as a top 10 defense in 2021 after adding some much-needed pass rush in the draft.

2021 Outlook:
They may have found the missing piece in Carson Wentz, who will try and do what Andrew Luck and Philip Rivers couldn't: Make it to the Super Bowl. Carson has struggled with injuries in the past but all of that now behind him, and he will need to stay on the field if this team is going to have the success that matches its immense talent on the roster. Fantasy owners are obviously frustrated with Carson and probably very apprehensive of making him their QB1, even in 1QB leagues. However, he's a steal in 1QB league drafts, and in 2QB/Superflex leagues, everyone will value him as a mid-QB2, so jump on that and get ready for your SuperFlex QB2 to wind up giving you QB1 value. The bottom line here: Owning Wentz, Taylor, or Pittman (or even all 3) is a very sneakily good game plan on your part.

Jacksonville Jaguars Fantasy Preview

Key losses: Doug Marrone (HC)
The Jags, for the most part, either bring every key player back for 2021 or add critical players. This alone is a good thing for the team as a whole. The only significant loss is former HC Doug Marrone. So why is this their top loss? Because bad play-calling and, well, overall bad play should be a thing of the past with Urban Meyer now in town.

Key additions: Shaq Griffin (CB), Marvin Jones (WR), Urban Meyer (HC)
The biggest addition this offseason for the Jags is, without a doubt, QB Trevor Lawrence whom they drafted No. 1 overall. That will make the biggest difference, and pairing Urban Meyer with Trevor could change this franchise for the better for years and years to come. The offense should immediately be one of the most interesting to watch in 2021. Marvin Jones will join D.J. Chark on the outside in 2-wide sets, and we can expect a ton of vertical, downfield fireworks with Lawrence as the triggerman. In addition, Griffin signed a 3-year, $40M deal and will get to play across from shutdown corner C.J. Henderson.

Drafted Players of Fantasy Note: Trevor Lawrence (QB), Travis Etienne (RB)

Trevor Lawrence, regardless of head coach, immediately injects a ton of life into this offense. He's a dual-threat, athletic QB with a great arm, great accuracy, and the ability to escape and extend plays. Pairing with Trevor in the backfield is his Clemson teammate Travis Etienne. A homerun-hitting tailback who is tough to bring down and sheds tackles like snakeskin. The dynamic nature of the offense on paper is enough to entice anyone.

Fantasy Impact:

As I've mentioned a few times already, adding Trevor will ignite this passing attack and send it soaring to a level we haven't seen from this franchise since the Jimmy Smith days. So, no need to rehash this. The running game is where things get interesting. James Robinson isn't going anywhere, even with the selection of Travis in the 1st round. Remember Rashaad Penny's pick by the Seahawks in the 1st round and how most people thought it was a death blow to Chris Carson? I think we're going to see something similar. I believe Travis will be heavily involved, but I do not think James Robinson's value is dead. He will still be a heavy contributor, even if it's not in an RB1 capacity. Urban may be trying to replicate the Chubb-Hunt combo we've seen in Cleveland, and if so, I want a piece of it. While everyone is clamoring over Etienne and letting Robinson slip too far, I would recommend jumping all over Robinson for immense value.

Offensive outlook:

As mentioned, the offense will see a vast increase in productivity in both fantasy and real life. It should be one of the more fun offenses to watch and keep tabs on as the season continues, and when we're all watching NFL RedZone on Sundays, there's going to be a lot more firepower when the Jags show up on your screen. I would tentatively expect Trevor Lawrence to be in the high-end QB2-low end QB1 range. It also wouldn't surprise me if he's a QB1 all season long. The Jags were 28th in the league in total offense in 2020. They will be significantly better in 2021 under Lawrence & Urban, and they may wind up as the most significant turnaround offense this season.

Defensive outlook:

The offseason additions of Shaq Griffin & Tyson Alualu should help this defense avoid last year's 31st ranked finish. They still need more pieces to prevent giving up so many points and yards to their opponents, but Griffin, more than anything, should assist in that area along with the return of their young stud CB C.J. Henderson.

2021 Outlook:

We can all enjoy a new, exciting offense under Urban Meyer, but when it comes to team success in the standings, things aren't likely to change much in Year 1. So from a fantasy perspective, there's only a "Big 4" to be concerned with: Lawrence, Chark, Robinson, and Etienne. If you're able to snag any of these four players, I believe you'll be plenty satisfied with what you get regarding where you're likely to be able to get them.

Houston Texans Fantasy Preview

Key losses: J.J. Watt (DE), Will Fuller (WR), DeShaun Watson (?) (QB), Bill O'Brien (HC)

The Texans lost LB Benardrick McKinney when they traded him to Miami for DE Shaq Lawson, but McKinney was never really an impact player. J.J. Watt, on the other hand? Yeah, it's safe to say he was an impact player. Watt was released in February, clearing $17.5M in cap space for a team that seems like they are in rebuild mode, prompting the trade for Shaq Lawson, a perennial underperformer. Will Fuller also departs to Miami via FA, leaving a hole at outside WR that will initially be Keke Coutee's job to fill across from Brandin Cooks. As of this writing, Watson is facing a flurry of sexual assault accusations, and it's unsure if he'll play in 2021 (or ever again if allegations are found to be true). The Texans already weren't a good football team, but losing Watson takes them out of the running for any competitiveness the fans could hope for. Perhaps new HC David Culley has some ideas to turn that around following the firing of crash-and-burn HC Bill O'Brien...about the only good thing to happen to the Texans this offseason.

Key additions: Mark Ingram (RB), Tyrod Taylor (QB), Phillip Lindsay (RB)

The Texans (more notably Bill O'Brien) stupidly traded WR DeAndre Hopkins for RB David Johnson last season. That experiment failed miserably, and now we see Mark Ingram join the fold who should be the favorite for early-down & goal-line work and could provide some sneaky high-end RB2 value this season. However, Phillip Lindsay departed Denver to join Ingram and Johnson in the backfield. We all know Lindsay can play and can do it all. He's likely to be second on the totem pole in touches for that backfield, but his fantasy value likely takes a significant hit as he'll be playing for a bad football team in a 3-man committee backfield. Tyrod Taylor looks to be the starter at QB right now while figuring out what the hell will happen with Watson. Not a great outlook for the Texans' offense.

Drafted Players of Fantasy Note: Davis Mills (QB), Nico Collins (WR), Brevin Jordan (TE)

Jordan isn't likely to provide much fantasy value (barring injuries) in 2021. Still, he needs to be on your radar in dynasty drafts as his only real competition for TE targets in the underwhelming Jordan Akins. Nico Collins enters an excellent spot with all the opportunity to climb the WR depth chart ladder. He's a talented, physical receiver with good speed and great size and was held back considerably by bad all-around QB play up in Michigan. His QB play won't improve much in Houston unless Watson plays, but he still has an excellent opportunity to see some meaningful targets. He's my favorite rookie WR to snag in the late 2nd round in rookie drafts. Davis Mills could have been a 1st rounder next year had he stayed in school, but he lands in a spot that could potentially see him make starts as early as this season if Tyrod Taylor plays poorly or gets injured. He's typically available in the 3rd round of SuperFlex rookie drafts and even later in 1QB rookie drafts.

Fantasy Impact:

The entire fantasy outlook for the Texans is bleak at best right now. No DeShaun Watson is a death sentence for HC David Culley's first season as head man. WR1 Brandin Cooks' outlook isn't nearly what it could be as the top guy with Watson, as Tyrod's ceiling, as we've seen plenty of times already, is pretty low as a passer. The only player on this entire team that I'm interested in owning this year is Mark Ingram, and even that is a dicey play, but the fact that you can get him so late in drafts is the only reason you'll want to take a shot as a depth piece on your bench. No one on this team will be a WR1, likely with or without Watson, and WR2 is probably even too optimistic. There isn't anything to like about this team in 2021 without Watson, and even with Watson, he may be the only thing to enjoy at that point. To me, even though Watson is going super late in drafts, it's not worth drafting him as your QB1 banking on him playing. If you select him, make sure it's your QB3 in Superflex or QB2 in 1QB leagues. It's not a dice you want to roll with the seriousness of the accusations and no end to this saga insight.

Offensive outlook:

Much like I stated above, there's nothing to get excited about without Watson. Ingram could provide some sneaky RB2 value, but that's about all you can hope for in this offense at this point. If Watson somehow can put all of this behind him and get the green light to play in 2021, Cooks becomes a lot more viable of a fantasy WR, but outside of him, there's still nothing you should be doing backflips over here. The 13th ranked overall offense in 2020 looks to take a massive slide down the ranks in 2021.

Defensive outlook:

Houston had the 30th ranked defense in 2020, and that was with J.J. Watt playing all 16 games. Without Watt and no impact defensive players drafted before the 5th round, this defense looks to be in dire straits heading into the season. They will likely be even worse than last season, and this unit is in even worse shape than the offense is.

2021 Outlook:

Last in the division. Top 3 draft pick. There you go, that's my outlook for the Texans. They would be lucky to avoid this prediction even with Watson. There's just nothing positive to take away from this team going into the 2021 season. Hell, it wasn't that long ago that we were talking about Watson wanting to be traded and not being on the roster at all. The bottom line, they won't be any good, and they're entirely too risky to roll the dice on almost any of their players being on your team this year. My advice? Just stay away altogether.

AFC WEST

Chris McConnell

Kansas City Chiefs Fantasy Preview

Key losses: Eric Fisher (OT)
Kansas City essentially replaced Eric Fisher after the Chiefs traded with the Ravens to acquire Orlando Brown, arguably upgrading the OL even more. More time for Pat to throw. Oh, boy.

Key additions: Orlando Brown (OT)
Orlando Brown joins the fold at offensive line and is easily the most significant addition this offseason. The O-line improved, and they fortified it a bit more in the draft. They hope the moves will help improve the blocking for Clyde Edwards-Helaire, who struggled when the field shrunk between the tackles.

Drafted Players of Fantasy Note: No drafted players of fantasy note

Fantasy Impact:
Do I need to read this story to you again? I mean, you know how it ends: With a top 3 offense in the NFL as long as the triplets (Mahomes, Kelce, and Hill) are all healthy. All three will be in tier 1 of their respective divisions and be reliable as hell week in and week out. You can't go wrong with drafting all three if you choose to. I'd probably suggest doing so. Sammy Watkins's departure opens up a massive opportunity for Mecole Hardman to turn into a reliable WR2 for fantasy. However, he's probably still not someone you want to be starting every week of the season.

Offensive outlook:
Again, the offense won't skip a beat. They returned nearly every one of relevance on the No. 1 overall offense in the league last season. They even got better with the offseason's offensive line upgrades. They'll pick right back up where they left off in 2020 and be back in the AFC's driver seat for another Super Bowl appearance.

Defensive outlook:
The Chiefs' defense was average as they ranked 16th in the league. But, of course, when your offense is as good as KC's is, you don't exactly need a top-flight defense...or do you? Tom Brady certainly proved that KC's dynamic offense wasn't going to be enough. Oddly, no significant defensive additions were made to the defense so far this offseason, but there's still time for that to change before the season. If the Chiefs roll into 2021 with what they have now, this season could have a similar ending as we saw back in February.

2021 Outlook:
As stated, this team will run through the AFC (for the most part) yet again, barring injuries. They're the Super Bowl favorite in the AFC again, and rightly so. However, I can pretty much sum up the Chief's 2021 fantasy outlook with the following: A QB1, a TE1, a WR, and an RB that could end up as an RB1. What else needs to be said?

Los Angeles Chargers Fantasy Preview

Key losses: Mike Pouncey (C), Casey Hayward (CB), Trai Turner (G)
Once one of the league's best CBs from 2016-2019, Casey Hayward was released, clearing nearly $10M in cap space and was even more expendable due to the play of Micahel Davis, who is now the Bolt's top outside cover corner. Of course, losing Turner and Pouncey on the OL hurts, but they drafted Rashawn Slater, who was arguably the best OL in the draft and will be tasked with making sure Justin Herbert stays upright.

Key additions: Jared Cook (TE)
#FreeDonaldParham.We all watched Donald Parham dominate at TE for the Dallas Renegades of the XFL. He's shown some flashes of that same ability in some tiny action he got for LAC in 2020 but hasn't yet been unleashed. Let's hope that changes, but it looks like it won't be in 2021. Jared Cook was signed to a 1-year deal and is locked in as the starter for now. Jared caught 7 TDs last season on 504 yards receiving. Those numbers are attainable in a Chargers offense where TEs combined for a 21.4% target share in 2020, and with Hunter Henry no longer in the fold, that alone frees up 93 targets that are now up for grabs. Couple that with Herbert, who is now coming off a great rookie season, and Cook could end up in the TE1 range. But still, can we please #FreeDonaldParham?

Drafted Players of Fantasy Note: Josh Palmer (WR), Tre McKitty (TE)
Josh Palmer and Tre McKitty were drafted in Round 3 of the draft, but they aren't fantasy relevant for 2021. If injuries occur at either position, you'll want to have them on your in the chamber just in case, but other than that, fantasy managers can ignore them outside of deep dynasty leagues for now.

Fantasy Impact: Justin Herbert. That's who it's all about. Justin was excellent last season, throwing for over 4,000 yards with 30 TDs and 10 INTs. We're all expecting an even better, more refined season this year, and he can deliver that. LAC is going to be a tough team to beat. Austin Ekeler returns as the undisputed workhorse RB1 for LAC and will probably remain in the expected top 6 for PPR RBs. Josh Kelley and Justin Jackson aren't that good, so Austin should have as much work as he can handle this season. Keenan Allen is a WR1, and that's a surprise to no one, but perhaps in Justin's second year, he can make a more consistent WR out of BMW (Big Mike Williams). One thing is for sure: This offense is going to be electric (pun fully intended).

Offensive outlook:
The offense should be back in the top 10 in 2021 (9th in 2020), but a lot will be dependent on the offensive line, which was the problem last year and was what they addressed in the first round by drafting Rashawn Slater. If the OL holds, this offense has the upside to be top 5 in the NFL while they trot out their fantasy QB1, RB1, and WR1.

Defensive outlook:
The Chargers' top 10 defense returns most of those responsible for that finish in 2020. They also add CB Asante Samuel Jr., whom they stole in the 2nd round of the draft. They're going to need all the help they can get and remain healthy while going up against Mahomes, the Raiders' offensive speed, and a Broncos team that could end up trading for Aaron Rodgers by the time the season starts.

2021 Outlook:
The Chargers finished 7-9 last season but ended the year on a four-game winning streak. They'll be the favorites to finish second in the division, and rightfully so. A team trotting out a top 10 offense and likely top 10 defense will need a lot to go wrong to not compete for a playoff spot. Don't be shy to make Herbert, Ekeler, and Allen 3 of the first players off the board at their position this season. Additionally, if you decide to put them all on your team, I won't be mad at you. That's a deadly trio.

Denver Broncos Fantasy Preview

Key losses: A.J. Bouye (CB), Jurrell Casey (DT)
Denver released A.J. to clear $13M in cap space, but it's not a significant loss as Bouye missed seven games due to a shoulder injury, concussion, and 6-game suspension. Casey, a 5-time pro bowler, was released to clear $11M in cap space but only appeared in 3 games in 2020. So, in other words, some enormous losses for the Broncos this offseason.

Key additions: Teddy Bridgewater (QB), Ronald Darby (CB)

The 27-year-old Darby signed a 3-year, $30M deal to fill a big need in the secondary for Denver. However, he's always been a bit of a roller-coaster type of player on the field, so it's not wise to rely on consistency. Drafting CB Patrick Surtain II, arguably the best CB in the draft is the second step in making sure Denver's secondary isn't nearly as leaky as it was in 2020. Teddy is the story here, though, as he was acquired by the Broncos in exchange for a 6th round pick and will compete to be the starting QB.

Drafted Players of Fantasy Note: Javonte Williams (RB)

Oh boy, do I love this move! Javonte slid to the 2nd round, and while I'm the chairman of the #RBDM (running backs don't matter) movement, that's only relevant for real life. They invested high draft capital in drafting a do-it-all RB to pair with Melvin Gordon, who is on his last leg. It's painfully apparent to anyone that watched Melvin towards the end of 2020 that he doesn't have it anymore, and he's about to expire. Javonte is my 2nd ranked RB in this rookie class for dynasty leagues (behind Najee Harris), and don't be afraid (in fact, feel encouraged) to draft him before Travis Etienne. Williams will be involved from Day 1 and, in my opinion, should take over as the starter shortly after week 8, if not earlier. Williams may not reach workhorse RB1 status in 2021, but he's in as sexy a situation as any and is an excellent target in the top 7 of your rookie drafts, even in Superflex leagues.

Fantasy Impact:

Well, take everything you read here with a grain of salt until we know for sure that Aaron Rodgers won't be playing in Mile High this year. As of this writing, he still hasn't been traded and ultimately may not be. If Rodgers ends up in Denver, Courtland Sutton, Jerry Jeudy, and Noah Fant's value skyrockets, and you're probably looking at a WR1-WR2-TE1 triple finish in fantasy for these guys. Suppose it's Teddy or Drew under center; good luck. Of course, all of these guys are talented enough to produce and wind up in tier 1 of their fantasy positions by the season's end. However, it'll be a lot harder to do when dealing with the inconsistency and limitations that come along with Lock & Bridgewater. It's best to draft the entire passing game with expectations that they all wind up in tier 2 of their fantasy positions instead. In Superflex drafts, do what you can to avoid being stuck with Teddy or Drew as your QB2.

Offensive outlook:

Denver was 23rd in the league in total offense last year, and while the injury to Sutton didn't help matters, they still indeed wouldn't have been any better than 20th. This offense for 2021 hinges on whether or not they can put together a deal for Aaron Rodgers after whiffing on so many QBs in the post-Peyton Manning era. Teddy & Drew won't do much to increase production for anyone on offense than what they did last year, so, unfortunately, it's probably the smart bet to not expect anything special from this team in reality or fantasy. Regardless, Javonte Williams is the story for now and the one intriguing piece I want to own everywhere I can in dynasty leagues.

Defensive outlook:

21st in total defense is the biggest reason why they added Ronald Darby and drafted Patrick Surtain. This team has got to stop the bleeding in the passing game, and these two may be the tandem to get that job done. The offense should be good enough to keep them competitive if the defense can stop opposing offenses from lighting them up. All in all, the AFC West should be one of the most competitive divisions in the NFL in 2021.

2021 Outlook:

Odds are, we're looking at another missed playoff season for the Broncos that show an improved defense and a slightly improved offense. But in all reality, the Chiefs, Chargers, and Raiders will make life difficult in the division for one another, and the Broncos will likely draw the shortest straw in that aspect. There could be some fantastic storylines with this team and its player development as the season goes along. But in regards to the playoffs and a Super Bowl, those are likely a true QB away. A QB like, oh, I don't know...Aaron Rodgers.

Las Vegas Raiders Fantasy Preview

Key losses: No key offseason losses

Key additions: John Brown (WR), Kenyan Drake (RB), Willie Snead (WR)
The Raiders added to receiving corps signings two solid lid-lifters in John Brown and Willie Snead. However, only John Brown should be impactful from a fantasy standpoint and shove a dagger into the value of Henry Ruggs. Kenyan Drake has been underutilized in Miami and then went to Arizona was mismanaged there as well, as, toward the end of his tenure in the desert, we saw Drake get almost wholly taken out of the receiving game, which is inexplicable. Drake, without a doubt, harms the value of Josh Jacobs, and it's a clear indicator that Gruden & Co. are not keen on keeping Josh Jacobs as a workhorse. Josh should still handle most early downs and goal-line work, but much of his receiving work is likely to slide over to Kenyan.

Drafted Players of Fantasy Note:
None of the players drafted by the Raiders will provide anything of fantasy note. Each pick was either on the offensive or defensive line.

Fantasy Impact:
This offense is only going to be as strong as Derek Carr allows it to be. Darren Waller is still the focal point and is the straw that stirs the drink in the passing game. John Brown was signed in March, but there was no considerable addition to the passing game that will take targets away from Waller even with him. He will remain a top-flight TE1 with no shortage of targets to work with. Draft him accordingly. The John Brown addition likely does a lot more to harm the value of fellow speedster Henry Ruggs. Ruggs isn't the type of receiver that will garner a large target load. This was the main reason I wasn't interested in drafting him last year, regardless of league format. The small number of targets he receives per game is now going to be impacted by John Brown. My advice? Sell your Henry Ruggs shares while you still can. Josh Jacobs is likely no longer in the RB1 conversation, but he should still offer RB2 solid value as the second RB you draft for your team, but the addition of Kenyan Drake should not be understated.

Offensive outlook:
Again, the offense will be as good as Derek Carr allows it to be. There are concerns on the OL, but the Raiders did spend 1st round capital on Alex Leatherwood, who, while many don't like the pick, will be tasked with helping turn this OL around and keep Carr upright and sure up the trenches for Josh & Kenyan. The Raiders lost no one of relevance to the 8th ranked offense in the league last year, and that's excellent news. This is an offense to keep an eye on as they could take it to the next level with Brown and Drake joining the fray and if Jacobs stays healthy. They don't exactly have that "alpha" WR1, and that seems to be the only thing they're missing, but for now, Waller has filled that role admirably for the last couple of seasons.

Defensive outlook:
Why did the Raiders spend almost every draft pick on defense? Because they needed to. This unit was ranked 25th in the league last season and was the sole reason this squad didn't win 10+ games. Another 8-8 record won't be good enough, and no matter how good Carr plays, he would likely be the scapegoat and be removed as the starter in 2022. But one step at a time. If a couple of these offseason defensive additions (including 2nd round pick Trevon Moehrig) play well enough, the Raiders could be in playoff contention in 2021.

2021 Outlook:
Sure, the Raiders could be in playoff contention this season, but the real problem will be their division-mates. They aren't topping the Chiefs, so the best they can hope for is a wild card spot, but an imposing Chargers squad is going to make it difficult on them, and as of this writing, Aaron Rodgers hasn't been traded to Denver...yet. If he is, that may all but seal the hopes of the Raiders' playoff hopes this season. Odds are, the Raiders will yet again be a good, not great, competitive team that challenges for 8-10 wins but falls short due to defensive woes and division competitiveness.

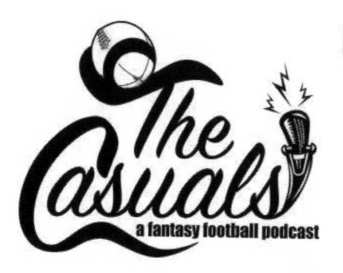

Home of the Lottery League!

Designed to interest the Casual. Adapted to challenge the Pro. Come test your luck to see if you have what it takes to prevail against even odds!

The interactive Fantasy Football experience you have been waiting for! Come join in on the fun and shenanigans with 4 not-so professional Fantasy Football pretend-experts!

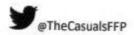 @TheCasualsFFP

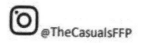 @TheCasualsFFP

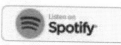 The Casuals FFP

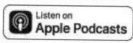 Listen on Apple Podcasts

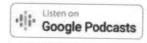 Listen on Google Podcasts

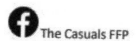 Listen on Spotify

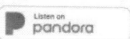 Listen on pandora

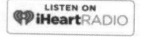 Listen on amazon music

LISTEN ON iHeartRADIO

NFC EAST

Chris Meaney

Dallas Cowboys Fantasy Preview

KEY LOSSES: Sean Lee (LB), Antwaun Woods (DT), Andy Dalton (QB), Cameron Erving (LG), Chidobe Awuzie (CB)

KEY ADDITIONS: Keanu Neal (LB), Tarell Bashman (DE), Dan Quinn (DC)

OFFSEASON FANTASY IMPACT:
Dak Prescott signing a four-year, $160m deal was the biggest offseason move for the Dallas Cowboys. This offense was cooking last season before Prescott suffered a season-ending ankle injury in Week 5. Dak had 1,856 passing yards (371.2/G) and was on pace to set the single-season yardage record. He had 12 total touchdowns (nine passing) and two four-touchdown games in his first five games (mostly four). The Cowboys averaged 34 points per game over Dak's first four contests of 2020.

NFL DRAFT PICKS OF FANTASY IMPACT: Micah Parsons, LB (Penn State); Simi Fehoko, WR (Stanford)
The Cowboys didn't need a wide receiver but they drafted Fehoko anyway, but not before drafting six defensive players. Dallas is loaded on offense so Fehoko won't have much of an impact this season unless injuries force him into a role. The Cowboys traded back in the first round once cornerbacks Jayce Horn and Patrick Surtain II were selected, and they landed Micah Parsons with the 12th pick. Parsons will be a player in IDP formats, especially for those who have a rookie only draft coming up. Parsons racked up 191 tackles and 6.5 sacks in two years at Penn State.

OFFENSIVE OUTLOOK:
There's no reason to think this offense won't be one of the NFL's best as Prescott's expected to be cleared in time for training camp. Amari Cooper, CeeDee Lamb and Michael Gallup are all strong targets for Prescott, Blake Jarwin is expected to be ready for Week 1, the offensive line is healthy and the run game is strong.

Ezekiel Elliott had a down season, but five of his six rushing touchdowns came in the first five weeks of the campaign and 24 of his 52 catches came in games Dak started. Elliott averaged 72.8 rushing yards and 107.8 total yards per game with Prescott and 61 rushing yards and 77.8 total yards per game without him. Dak and Zeke have "bounce back" written all over them. In fact, Prescott is favored to win the Comeback Player of the Year award.

DEFENSIVE OUTLOOK:
The defense improved throughout 2020 but they allowed the fifth-most points (29.6 per game), the second-most rushing yards (158.3 per game) and the 10th-most yards (386.4 per game). They let multiple defensive players walk through free agency and selected a defensive player with their first six picks. Dallas took three cornerbacks, including Kelvin Joseph with the 44th pick who has the skills to be a solid CB1 in the league. Maybe Dallas' biggest offseason move was the hiring of Dan Quinn to take over the defense. Coming with him from Atlanta is Keanu Neal who will reportedly switch from safety to weakside linebacker. Quinn will be tested as the Cowboys play five of last year's top seven passing offenses from last season.

2021 TEAM OUTLOOK:
The Cowboys have a 9.5 win total and are +125 favorites to win the NFC East. They have a top five offense and you can make the case they have a bottom 10 defense which usually results in fantasy gold. They'll play in plenty of fun games in 2021 and if you want a piece of their offense you're going to have to pay for it. Prescott is being drafted as a top five quarterback, his top two weapons in Amari Cooper and CeeDee are going inside the top 15 at the position, with the only discount coming at running back with Ezekiel Elliott. Don't let anyone tell you Zeke isn't a

top 10 RB or a strong pick at the end of the first. The defense is better but the offense will still be forced to put up points so get shares of this offense where you can.

New York Giants Fantasy Preview:

KEY LOSSES: Golden Tate (WR), Wayne Gallman (RB), Kevin Zeitler (RG), Dalvin Tomlinson (IDL)

KEY ADDITIONS: Kenny Golladay (WR), Kevin Rudolph (TE), Devontae Booker (RB), John Ross (WR), Adoree' Jackson (CB), Ifeadi Odenigbo (EDGE)

OFFSEASON FANTASY IMPACT:
The Giants spent money on both sides of the ball during free agency but Kenny Golladay was their biggest addition. The true X-receiver signed a five-year, $72M deal with the Giants ($40M guaranteed). Sterling Shepard, Darius Slayton, Golden Tate and Evan Engram combined for nine touchdown receptions in 2020. Golladay was limited to five games last season, but he caught 11 touchdowns on 65 grabs in 2019 en route to his second straight 1,000 yard season. KG had 2,253 yards and 135 catches on 235 targets from 2018-2019. That's 7.5 targets per game which I believe is doable in New York, but there's a definite downgrade at QB from Matthew Stafford to Daniel Jones.

The Giants took a flier on John Ross and they drafted Kadarius Toney who will eventually be the team's full time starter in the slot. Kyle Rudolph is a two-time Pro Bowl tight end with steady hands. The former Viking has only dropped two of his 233 targets over the last four seasons, and he only has two fumbles on his NFL resume. Devontae Booker will compete for the backup role behind Saquon Barkley.

NFL DRAFT PICKS OF FANTASY IMPACT: Kadarius Toney (WR), Gary Brightwell (RB)
Reports suggest the Giants were ready to take DeVonta Smith with their 11th pick but the Eagles traded up with the Cowboys to select the wideout out of Alabama. New York traded back and selected wide receiver Kadarius Toney with the 20th pick. The former high school QB is extremely raw as a route runner as 70 of his 120 catches in four years at Florida came last season. Toney brings much-needed speed to the Giants and he's a stud in the YAC department so he could serve as a gadget option or return man. He may not have much redraft value in his first season but it's important to note that Sterling Shepard has missed 10 games in the past two seasons. Brightwell was hardly used in his three seasons at Arizona as his 100 touches in 2020 were a career high for him. Booker and Brightwell will give the Giants depth at the position should Barkley suffer another season-ending injury.

OFFENSIVE OUTLOOK:
Only the New York Jets scored fewer points and had fewer yards than the Giants last season. New York only mustered 17.5 points and 299.6 yards per game in 2020. Their 189.1 passing yards per contest ranked 29th as did their 3,336 receiving yards overall. Many were expecting a breakout season from Daniel Jones in 2020 and we didn't see it. You had to pay a decent price for him last season but early indications are you don't in 2021 as he was QB21 on average in NFC drafts through the first two weeks of May. Jones has all the tools to succeed as a fantasy QB and he has upside due to his ability to run the football.

Barkley is on track to be ready for the start of the 2021 season as he recovers from a torn right ACL. Barkley suffered the injury in Week 2 and underwent successful surgery in October. The 24-year-old rushed for more than 1,000 yards in each of his first two seasons in the league, and he racked up 91 grabs as a rookie. It may seem like Saquon comes with a lot of risk on draft day but he's one of the few bell-cow backs in the league and he'll be gone within the first seven picks of most fantasy drafts.

DEFENSIVE OUTLOOK:
The Giants reeled in former first-round cornerback Adoree' Jackson in free agency to play opposite of James Bradberry. New York added three more corners in the draft as they selected Aaron Robinson in the third, Elerson

Smith in the fourth and Rodarius Williams in the sixth. It's an upgrade that was needed as they finished 22nd in Pass DVOA in 2020.

They were also able to retain DI Leonard Williams who is one of the game's best pass-rushers, and they drafted Azeez Ojulari who was PFF's highest-graded pass-rusher. New York allowed 28.2 points per game in 2019 which was the third-worst mark in the league, but last season they cut that number down to 22.3 which was the ninth best mark in the NFL. They could very well improve on that number yet again.

2021 TEAM OUTLOOK:
The New York Giants have a win total of 7 which I think is slightly unfair considering they won six games last season with Saquon Barkley only active for two contests. The over is very much in play with the NFL adding another game to its schedule. New York had a strong offseason as they brought in an alpha wideout in Golladay and they upgraded at cornerback with Jackson. They spent more money than any other team in the NFC East which doesn't always result in wins but they backed it up with a strong draft.

Philadelphia Eagles Fantasy Preview

KEY LOSSES: Carson Wentz (QB), Alshon Jeffery (WR), DeSean Jackson (WR), Jalen Mills (CB)

KEY ADDITIONS: Kerryon Johnson (RB), Joe Flacco (QB), Anthony Harris (DB)

OFFSEASON FANTASY IMPACT:
The Eagles weren't big players in free agency as they were up against the cap so they didn't bring any impactful names in. Their biggest move was trading Carson Wentz to the Indianapolis Colts after five seasons with the club. Wentz is reunited with Frank Reich who was the OC when the Eagles won the Super Bowl. The trade opens up the door for second-year player Jalen Hurts to be the starting QB for the Eagles. Philadelphia also moved on from Alshon Jeffery and DeSean Jackson as they look to get younger at the position.

NFL DRAFT PICKS OF FANTASY IMPACT: DeVonta Smith (WR), Kenneth Gainwell (WR), Landon Dickerson (C)
The Eagles have missed on so many wideouts over the years so they made a point in trading up to snag DeVonta Smith. Last year's Heisman Trophy winner joins his former Alabama teammate Jalen Hurts and he may just lead all rookie wideouts in targets. The Eagles cut Jeffery and Jackson, so there are plenty of targets available. Much has been made about Smith's weight but he's as complete as they come at the position and he's fresh off an 1856-yard season which saw him score 23 touchdowns on 117 catches. He has flex appeal with WR3 upside in year 1 and he's a strong get in dynasty leagues.

Kenneth Gainwell is a strong pass catching back that will cut into Boston Scott's role and potentially Miles Sanders' passing down work as the back struggled with drops in 2020. The selection of Gainwell and addition of Kerryon Johnson likely makes Sanders a fade when you consider the rushing ability of Hurts. Landon Dickerson doesn't have any fantasy appeal but he's a nice addition to an offensive line that was rattled with injuries last season.

OFFENSIVE OUTLOOK:
Heading into the offseason many wondered if it would be Doug Pederson or Carson Wentz's team in 2021 but the Eagles decided to move on from both. Philly shipped Wentz to Indianoplis, they hired Nick Sirianni as the head coach and Shane Steichen was brought in to be the OC. Sirianni served as the OC in Indy for the last three seasons and Steichen had the same role last season with the Chargers, but that was his first as a coordinator. There are plenty of questions heading into the season, but make no mistake about it Jalen Hurts will be Sirianni's starting quarterback. Hurts' rushing ability puts him in the QB1 conversation and I believe he has the upside to finish as a top 10 QB, despite the lack of weapons. Smith is a huge get, Jalen Reagor has the upside to be a FLEX, and Dallas Goedert has top five upside at the TE position. Zach Ertz remains on the roster for now, but he offered very little to Philadelphia when he was healthy.

Miles Sanders was limited to 12 games last season and failed to return a profit so he'll come with a discount in 2021. Fantasy owners screamed for more touches as Sanders' 5.3 YPC was the fourth best mark among running backs. Unfortunately for owners, he only averaged 13.6 touches per game and he struggled in the passing game. Will he get more touches under Sirianni? How often will Hurts steal touches from Sanders in the red zone? It's hard to tell but if Sanders falls outside the top 15 at the position, I'll be interested.

DEFENSIVE OUTLOOK:
The Eagles not only cleaned house on offense they did on defense as well as they hired Jonathan Gannon to replace long time defensive coordinator Jim Schwartz. Gannon served as the Colts' cornerbacks and defensive back coach for the last three years. The 38-year-old is the fourth-youngest DC in the NFL.

The Eagles secondary took a step forward last season with the addition of Darius Slay but they still finished 24th in Pass DVOA. There are still holes in the secondary but they used to be one of the worst units in the league, but in 2020 they ranked 18th in passing yards allowed per game (237.9). It was their rush defense that took a step back in 2020 as they coughed up the 10th most rushing yards per game (125.8). They allowed the third-fewest in 2019 and the seventh-fewest in 2018. They have players like Brandon Graham, Fletcher Cox and Derek Barnett who can get after the QB, but this is a middle-of-the-pack defense at best.

2021 TEAM OUTLOOK:
The Eagles have the lowest team implied total in the NFC EAST as it sits at 6.5. They have the easiest schedule based on last year's record but we know that's a misleading stat. All three teams improved in the division and the Eagles have games against Kansas City, Tampa Bay, San Francisco, New Orleans and the Chargers. There are still plenty of talented players on this roster and it starts with the offensive line.

Last year they were behind the eight ball with injuries to Brandon Brooks and Andre Dillard to start the season followed by Lane Johnson among others. The Eagles had 11 different combinations on their o-line in their first 11 games, so finding some stability there will help this offense. The truth is, the schedule isn't easy and there's a lack of experience on the roster and in the coaching staff.

Washington Football Team Fantasy Preview

KEY LOSSES: Alex Smith (QB), Ronald Darby (CB), Kevin Pierre-Louis (LB), Ryan Kerrigan (EDGE)

KEY ADDITIONS: Ryan Fitzpatrick (QB), Curtis Samuel (WR), Adam Humphries (WR), Ereck Flowers (LG), William Jackson III (CB)

OFFSEASON FANTASY IMPACT:
Terry McLaurin dynasty owners had to be thrilled when Washington signed Ryan Fitzpatrick as he's had to deal with poor QB play since he entered the league. The 38-year-old certainly isn't the long term answer for Washington and they'll have to address the position through the draft at some point, but he's always been a solid fantasy QB because he's not afraid to push the ball down the field.

Washington also signed wideout Curtis Samuel who current head coach Ron Rivera drafted when he was with the Carolina Panthers. Samuel had a career-high 77 receptions, 851 yards and 200 rushing yards. He's one of the most versatile offensive weapons in the league, who found a home in the slot last season. This offense is on the rise, they'll be fun to watch and they won't have to score many points to win football games with as good as the defense is.

NFL DRAFT PICKS OF FANTASY IMPACT: Dyami Brown (WR), Dax Milne (WR), John Bates (TE)

Washington added more speed with Dyami Brown, who averaged 20 yards per reception in the last two seasons at North Carolina. His blazing speed is a big reason why he saw an averaged depth of target of 18.4 last season and 17.4 in 2019. While some may view him as a one-trick-pony, Brown has the ability to take one to the house on a slant. The third-round wideout is an underrated deep-ball specialist who could serve as a game-changer for Fitz and company.

OFFENSIVE OUTLOOK:

It may have taken longer than anticipated but Washington is starting to build an explosive unit on offense. They absolutely hit on Terry McLaurin in 2019 and they followed it up in 2020 with their selection of Antonio Gibson who finished with 795 rushing yards (247 receiving) and 11 touchdowns. Samuel adds another element in the passing game which they didn't have last season and they so desperately needed.

Logan Thomas had a very solid season as he caught 72 balls and scored six touchdowns, but this offense needed more as ranked 30th in total yards per game (317.3), 24th in passing yards (216.6), 26th in rushing (100.7) and 25th in scoring (20.9 PPG). I love all of their weapons and they should be targets of yours on draft day. Fitzpatrick finished seventh in yards per attempt last season at 7.8 and we all know he can push the ball down the field to some of these weapons on offense. He won't need to throw the ball 40 plus times in this offense but he still has all the makings of a strong QB2 or bye week replacement in fantasy.

DEFENSIVE OUTLOOK:

Washington had one of the best defenses in the league last season and they were led by 2020 NFL Defensive Rookie of the Year Chase Young. In 2019, Washington coughed up the fifth-most yards, the second-most rushing yards and they only had three wins. Young helped the Football Team finish fifth in points per game (20.6) and second in passing yards per game (191). They were one of only three teams (Rams and Steelers) to allow fewer than 200 passing yards, and the Los Angeles Rams were the only team to allow fewer total yards and passing yards than WFT. Young, Montez Sweat and Da'Ron Payne will be a problem for opposing teams yet again.

2021 TEAM OUTLOOK:

Washington surprised everyone last season as they went from picking second in the NFL draft to winning the NFC East at 7-9. Say what you want about the division but the defense is legit and if they had a capable QB they may have made some noise in the playoffs as they lost 31-23 to the eventual Super Bowl champs. Washington checks in with a win total of eight which is a fair number given the extra game and a defense that will keep them in most games.

NFC NORTH

NATE HAMILTON

Green Bay Packers Fantasy Preview

KEY LOSSES: Aaron Rodgers? (QB), Jamaal Williams (RB)
KEY ADDITIONS: Blake Bortles (QB), Amari Rodgers (WR), Aaron Jones (RB)

OFFSEASON FANTASY IMPACT:

What an offseason it has been for the Green Bay Packers. Pretty much everyone (including myself) expected Aaron Jones to move on, instead, he was signed to another four years in Green Bay. As a result, the hype for running back A.J. Dillon was quickly put on ice. Most teams were excited for day one of the NFL draft, but it turned into a PR nightmare for the Packers as word got out in regards to Aaron Rodgers' discontent with the organization.

There is still plenty of uncertainty surrounding the Packers' future. They signed veteran quarterback, Blake Bortles as a precautionary measure. It's clear, the front office and coaching staff are not convinced that their 2020 1st round pick, Jordan Love is the answer at quarterback. If Aaron Rodgers remains with Green Bay for the 2021 season, everyone can breathe a sigh of relief in regards to their fantasy assets. If Rodgers moves on, it will have many positive and negative implications depending on his landing spot.

NFL DRAFT PICKS OF FANTASY IMPACT:

The Green Bay Packers spent a 3rd round (85th overall) pick on Clemson wide receiver, Amari Rodgers. Was this finally a move to make Aaron Rodgers happy with another offensive weapon? Is the gesture enough or too late? Either way, the addition of Amari Rodgers provides a great slot wideout to target for whoever is at quarterback in 2021. Even if Aaron Rodgers doesn't return, expect Amari to see a fair share of targets from either Blake Bortles or Jordan Love. He could end up being the comfortable, easy target out of the slot for a quarterback not named Aaron Rodgers.

OFFENSIVE OUTLOOK:

The outlook for the Packers' offense truly hinges on Aaron Rodgers. If he's back, the Packers will be among the top offenses in the league. If he's gone, growing pains will be had. Davante Adams has already spoken out and said he'd have to do some "extra thinking" on his future with the Packers if Rodgers were to leave.

Quarterback drama aside, the Packers have one of the best wide receivers in the game and a decent complimentary group. Running back, Aaron Jones will be ready to carry this team if need be, now that he's been signed to a four-year $48M deal with the Packers. Every offensive weapon will have to step up and make the most of the situation regardless of who is under center Week 1 of the 2021 season.

DEFENSIVE OUTLOOK

The Packers were already a top-10 defense in 2020, but that didn't stop them from adding to it in this year's NFL draft. They invested their 1st round pick (29th overall) in Georgia cornerback, Eric Stokes. Pairing Stokes with Jaire Alexander is going to create major problems for opposing offenses.

As promising as their defense is looking for the 2021 season, they too, are impacted by the Aaron Rodgers drama. Their jobs will become increasingly difficult throughout the season if their star quarterback isn't on the field extending the time of possession.

2021 TEAM OUTLOOK:

The 2021 outlook for the Green Bay Packers is simple. If Aaron Rodgers is the starting quarterback, everything remains status quo. If not, we will all have to re-evaluate the value of the fantasy assets on the Packers and whichever team Aaron Rodgers decides to sign with. If for some reason Aaron Rodgers decides to retire, we will be saying goodbye to one of the best quarterbacks the NFL has ever seen.

Chicago Bears Fantasy Preview

KEY LOSSES: N/A
KEY ADDITIONS: Justin Fields (QB), Andy Dalton (QB), Damien Williams (RB)

OFFSEASON FANTASY IMPACT:

Another NFC North team with quarterback concerns. The Bears signed veteran quarterback, Andy Dalton as they declined Mitchell Trubisky's fifth-year option. It appeared the Bears had little to no urgency in upgrading at quarterback until word got out that they reportedly offered the Seahawks three first-round picks, a 2021 third-round pick, and a couple of players. Unfortunately, for the Bears, Pete Carroll rejected the offer.

NFL DRAFT PICKS OF FANTASY IMPACT:

The Bears restored the faith of their fanbase when they moved up nine spots in the 2021 NFL draft to get Ohio State quarterback, Justin Fields with the 11th overall pick. As of now, the Bears are preparing to have Andy Dalton as their Week 1 starter, but a lot can change by then. Let's hope for fantasy-football-sake, Justin Fields starts sooner rather than later.

Regardless of who will be the quarterback, he will have decent protection. The Bears addressed offensive line needs with their round two and round five picks. This spells good things for the offensive fantasy players in Chicago for the 2021 season.

OFFENSIVE OUTLOOK:

There have been a lot of changes for the Bears' offense this season. They have upgraded their quarterback position (once Fields is named the starter), Tarik Cohen is returning from injury, they signed running back Damien Williams and focused heavily on offense in the draft.

Allen Robinson signed his franchise tag and will make $18M in 2021. David Montgomery will look to continue rolling after coming off an amazing season as the RB4 in fantasy football. The return of Cohen will certainly impact Montgomery's target/reception numbers.

DEFENSIVE OUTLOOK

The Bears are not world-beaters at defense and they got worse this offseason. They allowed Kyle Fuller to walk and "replaced" him with Desmond Trufant. A significant downgrade at cornerback.

Chicago could have used improvements via draft picks, however, Chicago decided to focus on offense in the 2021 draft. They did draft two defensive players but used their last two picks (228 & 250 overall) of the draft to address the need.

2021 TEAM OUTLOOK:

There are some exciting pieces on the Bears roster from a fantasy football standpoint. Allen Robinson will benefit from an upgrade at quarterback. Tight end, Cole Kmet could end up being a safety blanket for the rookie quarterback, Justin Fields. David Montgomery should be a value in 2021 fantasy drafts due to the return of Tarik Cohen and the addition of Damien Williams. Of course, all of these options come with risk as the Chicago Bears still have needs to be addressed if they want to be contenders.

Minnesota Vikings Fantasy Preview

KEY LOSSES: Kyle Rudolph (TE)

KEY ADDITIONS: Defense

OFFSEASON FANTASY IMPACT:

The Vikings haven't deviated from their 2020 fantasy weapons. Adding Kyle Rudolph as a "key loss" was strictly to call out Irv Smith's increased value. They have a well-rounded offense with some elite options for fantasy football. The Vikings have focused a lot on defense both in free agency and the NFL draft. The Vikings' fantasy-relevant players will hold value in 2021 with a major increase for Justin Jefferson.

NFL DRAFT PICKS OF FANTASY IMPACT:

Minnesota did not draft any fantasy-relevant options to impact the 2021 season. They are looking to the future at quarterback with Texas A&M, Kellen Mond using their second draft pick (66 overall) and a 4th-round running back (Kene Nwangwu, 119th overall pick). There would have to be an injury or performance issue from Kirk Cousins and pure devastation to the running back corps for either of these moves to have 2021 implications.

OFFENSIVE OUTLOOK:

I don't expect there to be significant changes to the fantasy outlook of Dalvin Cook, Kirk Cousins, or Adam Thielen in regards to where you should be drafting them. Justin Jefferson will likely cost you a 2nd-round to early 3rd-round pick and he's more than worth it. Some of you may want to take a chance on Irv Smith in the later rounds and I can't blame you. As much hate as Kirk Cousins gets, he produces for fantasy football and it may be time for Irv Smith to have a big impact in 2021.

DEFENSIVE OUTLOOK

As mentioned above, the Vikings made plenty of defensive moves this offseason. They have added some veterans to the mix including Xavier Woods, Patrick Peterson, Dalvin Tomlinson, and Mackensie Alexander. Getting older isn't best, but in this case, Minnesota needs leadership on defense.

2021 TEAM OUTLOOK:

This may seem a bit redundant in regards to my take on the Minnesota Vikings offense for 2021, but there just isn't any significant changes from 2020 to this season. A slight bump to Irv Smith especially in tight-end premium leagues and of course the elite status of wide receiver, Justin Jefferson.

If you play in any leagues that utilize team defenses, then the Vikings defense has certainly improved enough from last season for you to consider having them as your fantasy defense in 2021.

Detroit Lions Fantasy Preview

KEY LOSSES: Matthew Stafford (QB), Kenny Golladay (WR), Marvin Jones Jr. (WR)
KEY ADDITIONS: Jared Goff (QB), Breshad Perriman (WR), Tyrell Williams (WR), Jamaal Williams (RB)

OFFSEASON FANTASY IMPACT:

No question, the Detroit Lions have gone through more changes than any other team in the NFC North for the 2021 season. They no longer have Matthew Stafford at quarterback, instead, it will be former Los Angeles Rams quarterback, Jared Goff. A great Lions' wide receiver duo in Kenny Golladay and Marvin Jones Jr. also find themselves on new teams this year.

NFL DRAFT PICKS OF FANTASY IMPACT:
The Lions' new quarterback, Jared Goff will have some protection in the form of Penei Sewell. He was the best offensive lineman in the draft and the Lions utilized their #7 overall pick to draft him. Sewell will frustrate opposing defenses by giving his quarterback time to throw the ball and creating holes for D'Andre Swift and former Packers running back, Jamaal Williams. The Lions drafted USC wideout, Amon-Ra St. Brown with the 112th overall pick to add some depth to their depleted wide receiver corps.

OFFENSIVE OUTLOOK:
To say this offense will look much different in 2021 would be quite an understatement. They have a different quarterback and a different set of wide receivers with Breshad Perriman and Tyrell Williams leading the group. D'Andre Swift no longer has Adrian Peterson in the backfield and is expected to have his breakout season. A new coaching regime will be in effect as well which essentially hits a much-needed reset button on the franchise.

DEFENSIVE OUTLOOK
The Lions invested three of their first four draft picks on defensive assets. With Aaron Glenn officially the team's defensive coordinator, this defense will look much different than it did in 2020. Fans should be excited for the changes made this offseason. A productive defense will certainly help the offensive weapons by giving them more time of possession and opportunities.

2021 TEAM OUTLOOK:
I feel like this season can go one of two ways with no middle-ground for the Detroit Lions. All of the changes can come together and create a productive, winning culture or they continue with their woes of living at the bottom of the NFC North.

For fantasy football purposes, you should be able to attain most of the offensive assets in the later rounds. D'Andre Swift being the only outlier. Breshad Perriman showed an amazing quality as a WR1 in Tampa Bay when both Mike Evans and Chris Godwin were out due to injury. Tyrell Williams has also shown flashes in the past. Both Williams and Perriman have a shot to be the WR1 in an offense that will likely have to throw a ton in 2021.

NFC SOUTH

Lauren Carpenter

Tampa Bay Buccaneers Fantasy Preview

KEY LOSSES: LeSean McCoy (RB)

KEY ADDITIONS: Giovani Bernard (RB), C.J. Prosise (RB)

OFFSEASON FANTASY IMPACT: The Tampa Bay Buccaneers are primed to repeat their championship run to the Super Bowl again in 2021. The franchise made it a priority to bring back the team from last season, locking up QB Tom Brady, RB Leonard Fournette, and WR Chris Godwin. Practically the entire team is back, including Antonio Brown, who ran into some roadblocks in contract negotiations. McCoy remains a free agent after playing ten games and seeing 25 total touches in 2020.

The addition of Bernard to the RB room is interesting. While it may not be devastating to RBs Ronald Jones or Fournette, it's also not all that great for their fantasy production with only so many rush attempts to go around. It also doesn't bode well for second-year player Ke'Shawn Vaughn. Adding both Bernard and Prosise to the roster is another proverbial nail in the coffin regarding HC Bruce Arians' trust in the young running back.

Bernard has been with the Cincinnati Bengals since entering the league in 2009. Last season, with RB Joe Mixon sidelined with injury, Bernard rushed 124 times for 416 yards and three touchdowns. He also added 47 receptions on 59 targets for 355 yards and three touchdowns to his stat line. So, while he may not be a primary target for your team (unless you're in deeper leagues), he could affect just how much volume both Jones and Fournette see this year if they stay healthy.

NFL DRAFT PICKS OF FANTASY IMPACT: The Buccaneers don't have many holes to fill on their squad, so it's not surprising that their draft was pretty uneventful from a fantasy perspective. Nevertheless, they selected Florida's QB, Kyle Trask, in the 2nd Round to study behind both Tom Brady and Blaine Gabbert, and they also picked WR Jaelon Darden out of North Texas. With the quarterback (obviously) and so many receivers already solidified as champions, Trask and Darden likely won't see many offensive snaps. Still, Darden may be contributing to special teams with his speed and ability.

OFFENSIVE OUTLOOK: The Buccaneers are packed with studs (again), and it would behoove the fantasy manager to take a piece of this offense. In PPR scoring, Brady finished as the QB8, Mike Evans barely missed out of the top-10 as WR11, and TE Rob Gronkowski finished as the TE8. About the only position group that is the weakest in terms of fantasy are the running backs, with Jones finishing as the RB15. Still, if Jones falls in drafts or if Fournette and Bernard are available later, it would be difficult to pass up on a flex option out of those players. If healthy, Evans should continue to produce at a high level. Godwin should take a step forward, building his chemistry with Brady, and snagging a WR3 or WR4 such as Antonio Brown or even Scotty Miller or Tyler Johnson as a flyer late could be worth it.

DEFENSIVE OUTLOOK: Tampa didn't forget its defense when they scrambled to keep their dream team going for 2021. Ndamukong Suh, Shaquil Barrett, and Lavonte David (among others) were all re-signed to keep the streak alive. The Buccaneers DST finished as 9th best in 2020 with 15 interceptions, 48 sacks, 713 tackles, 15 fumbles, and averaging roughly 10 points a game. It won't just be the offensive pieces that are powerhouses in both real and fantasy football yet again in 2021.

2021 TEAM OUTLOOK: There is nothing on paper to show that the Buccaneers can't keep running the NFC South this year with a team that was just beginning to gel last season and won the Super Bowl anyway. This year may see the team and all of its fantasy-relevant positions explode right out of the gate instead of the sluggish start in 2020.

Carolina Panthers Fantasy Preview

KEY LOSSES: Teddy Bridgewater (QB), Curtis Samuel (WR), Mike Davis (RB)

KEY ADDITIONS: Sam Darnold (QB)

OFFSEASON FANTASY IMPACT: When it comes to offseason moves, the Panthers made a monumental one acquiring QB Sam Darnold from the Jets and offloading Teddy Bridgewater to the Broncos. After the draft, the Panthers exercised Darnold's fifth-year option, affirming their faith in the new quarterback.

NFL DRAFT PICKS OF FANTASY IMPACT: Terrace Marshall Jr. (WR), Chuba Hubbard (RB). The Panthers started their draft by addressing their needs at cornerback but took three offensive players following their 1st Round pick. So giving Darnold another weapon at receiver makes sense. Marshall was ranked third in the SEC for receiving touchdowns, ninth for touchdowns from scrimmage, and ninth for receiving. He will also be reunited with former LSU offensive coordinator Joe Brady.

The steal for Carolina was snagging Hubbard in the 4th Round out of Oklahoma State. This would be a little more exciting for fantasy managers if the Panthers didn't already have the best running back in football in Christian McCaffrey. If McCaffrey can stay healthy, Hubbard will likely have much less value in fantasy. However, if 2020 repeats itself, Hubbard could get a shot at the spotlight with Mike Davis now with the Falcons.

OFFENSIVE OUTLOOK: Seeing McCaffrey make some on-field magic this season will be a welcome relief for fantasy managers who will likely still draft him at the 1.01. Even adding Darnold as the new QB, make no mistake, this team's offense will still run through McCaffrey. WRs D.J. Moore and Robby Anderson are more intriguing this year with Darnold, and it will be interesting to see if he and Anderson can reignite some chemistry from their days with the Jets.

With Moore's talent, he can easily score WR1 weeks without the hefty draft capital and would be a solid WR2 for a lineup with massive upside. Anderson should be considered a WR3/Flex option without the consistency that Moore can provide. Darnold can be regarded as an asset in 2QB or Superflex leagues and could be an option to steam depending on the matchups.

Samuel's departure vacates 97 targets. Many of these are likely to go to both Moore and Anderson, but Marshal is an exciting look as a late-round flier who may be able to make an immediate impact this year as a rookie.

DEFENSIVE OUTLOOK: The Panthers had some severe needs on defense that they addressed during the draft. Their first overall pick with CB Jaycee Horn was a good start, but that's about it. Their defensive ranks are in the middle of the road and trending toward the bottom half. They could be a look to stream for fantasy but beware of their opponent's passing volume. The Panthers allowed the seventh-most attempts and sixth-most receptions in 2020.

2021 TEAM OUTLOOK: Darnold is a shiny new toy in Carolina, but it's still up in the air whether or not he is an upgrade at the QB position over Teddy Bridgewater. Their beleaguered offensive line will need to do a better job protecting their new quarterback and creating an opportunity for McCaffrey to go ham. Their future for real football is still pretty bleak, considering they are in the same division as the reigning Super Bowl champions in the Tampa Bay Buccaneers, who look primed to make a repeat run to the big game.

Atlanta Falcons Fantasy Preview

KEY LOSSES: Todd Gurley (RB), Ito Smith (RB)

KEY ADDITIONS: Mike Davis (RB)

OFFSEASON FANTASY IMPACT: The Falcons are in desperate need of a solid run game. Signing Mike Davis was a good start, but he may not be the kind of bell-cow running back we are used to seeing in an RB1. Davis benefited from a Chrisitan McCaffery injury in 2020 while with the Panthers but barely produced RB1 numbers. He rushed 165 times for only 642 yards and six touchdowns over 15 games while being the starter in 12 of them. He had 59 receptions on 70 targets for 373 yards and two receiving touchdowns. He was fifth in the league in targets among RBs and fourth in receptions finishing as the RB12 in PPR, scoring over 17 weeks.

NFL DRAFT PICKS OF FANTASY IMPACT: Kyle Pitts (TE). Labeled as a "unicorn," Pitts will make a big splash for the Falcons right out of the gate. He put up impressive numbers during his time at the University of Florida, including 43 receptions for 770 yards and 12 touchdowns last year in only eight games.

OFFENSIVE OUTLOOK: While the Falcons may lack the ground and pound type of running back like Derrick Henry, they benefit from adding another pass-catcher to the already high-passing style of offense. QB Matt Ryan had 628 pass attempts, which was fourth-highest in 2020, and that doesn't look like it's slowing down for 2021. WR Julio Jones has had an entire offseason to get healthy and hopefully return to elite status if he remains with the team. His age and injury history are a concern, but Atlanta also boasts 2020's breakout star, Calvin Ridley. Ridley not only led the NFL with over 2,000 air yards, but he also led the league with eight games of over 100 receiving yards. TE Hayden Hurst saw a career-high 88 targets in his first year in Atlanta after playing second-fiddle to Mark Andrews in Baltimore. Those targets translated to 56 receptions, 571 yards, and six touchdowns with a 63.6% catch rate.

New HC Arthur Smith will bring a new dynamic to the offense as a whole. He ran more 12-personnel than any other team in 2020 as the offensive coordinator for the Titans. That means there is one running back and two tight ends in the formation. Think Los Angeles Rams offense with Tyler Higbee and Gerald Everett. Not only does this add more weapons for Ryan, but it is good for both Pitts and Hurst as the two tight ends split on the field.

DEFENSIVE OUTLOOK: The Falcons' offense will remain pass-heavy, pass-early, and pass-because-we-are-playing from behind to win if they cannot shore up their defense. They allowed the fourth-most total yards per game with 398.4. Out of that total, they were dead last in passing yards allowed with 293.6 yards per game. Their run defense fared better in 2020, allowing the 6th fewest rushing yards per game with 91.3. Their DST averaged roughly 4.5 points per game and finished 24th depending on the individual league scoring, of course. The point is, they weren't perfect. They have added several young pieces to their defense, including new faces to their secondary, but they may need time to mature before they can gel and provide relief for Ryan and the offense.

2021 TEAM OUTLOOK: There isn't much about the Falcons (especially in PPR scoring) that makes me want to steer clear, except for Davis in standard or non-PPR scoring formats. This bodes well for fantasy, and snagging a piece of the offense would be a good idea, mainly if the capital isn't too steep. They may very well have two WR1 in Jones and Ridley, a TE1 in Pitts (and perhaps also Hurst), and an RB with top-10 weeks at the very least in Davis.

New Orleans Saints Fantasy Preview

KEY LOSSES: Drew Brees (QB), Emmanuel Sanders (WR), Jared Cook (TE)

KEY ADDITIONS: Nick Vannett (TE)

OFFSEASON FANTASY IMPACT: The Saints had quite an offseason heading into 2021. While it wasn't the number of players they lost, it all came down to losing the key offensive cog in QB Drew Brees. While Brees struggled down the stretch with his deeper passes and missed four games last season, he was still (and remains) a first-ballot Hall of Famer. That kind of loss is keen in a locker room. The Saints signed QB Jameis Winston to a one-year $12 million deal, and QB/TE Taysom Hill remains on the roster to compete for the job. However, when it comes to playing styles, Winston and Hill are practically the north and south pole. Additionally, with WR Emmanuel Sanders and TE Jared Cook both gone, some holes need to be filled and roles that players must step into.

Nick Vannett has jumped around the NFL from the Seahawks for three seasons, to Pittsburgh, back to Seattle, then to Denver, and is now in New Orleans. He is not a target-heavy tight end but has proven productive when he gets involved with a 71.4% catch rate out of 105 targets over his career.

NFL DRAFT PICKS OF FANTASY IMPACT: Ian Book (QB). The Saints were focused on their defense, which was already great, during the 2021 draft. As a result, they did not select anyone on offense until the 4th Round when they took Book then picked WR Kawaan Baker in the 7th Round. Book and Baker likely won't make an immediate impact for redraft in 2021, but Baker does have the opportunity to fill in where Sanders left off if he can make a name for himself to compliment Michael Thomas.

OFFENSIVE OUTLOOK: It's difficult to predict how the offense will shape up in 2021 if Winston is at the helm in New Orleans. He only played 47 snaps the entire year, which equated to 11 attempts, seven completions, and 75 yards. Ten of those attempts were Week 10 against San Francisco that resulted in six of those completions for 63 yards.

Even if Hill gets the nod in 2021, he only played a full-time quarterback in four games while the team historically used him as a swiss army knife in the red zone. However, Alvin Kamara managers will remember with distressing clarity Hill's effect on the RB's fantasy production in two out of the four weeks Hill started. In Week 12, Kamara finished as the RB36 in PPR scoring with only 48% of the snaps, 54 rushing yards, two targets, and one reception. Week 13 wasn't much better, but Hill eventually figured out that Kamara is good at catching a football and targeted him ten times in Week 14. Winston, however, managed to find Kamara four times for 52 yards in only 34 snaps while Hill had to take full games to get Kamara 53 receiving yards. Because Hill relies more on his legs and Winston on his arm (whether for better or ill), fantasy managers should hope for Winston to get the starting job while Saints fans of real football may want to lean on Hill.

The future looks a little brighter for Thomas this year if he can stay healthy. The absence of Cook and WR Sanders vacates a total of 142 targets up for grabs with no elite WR2 competition. WR Tre'Quan Smith will be on the roster for 2021, but he only saw 50 targets over 14 games while Thomas saw 55 targets in just seven.

DEFENSIVE OUTLOOK: The Saints, once again, have a high-powered DST unit. They have allowed the seventh-fewest passing yards (3,759) and fourth-fewest rushing yards (1,502) that results in the fourth-fewest total yards (4,974) in 2020. Their defense also tied for first in the league in interceptions with 18 and racked up 45 sacks, 653 tackles, and averaged the fifth-fewest points allowed per game at 21.1. They are on pace to repeat another excellent year on defense for fantasy, especially after selecting three defensive players in the first three rounds of the draft.

2021 TEAM OUTLOOK: Losing future hall of fame quarterback Drew Brees isn't ideal for the Saints' potential for a Super Bowl run, but there is no denying the weapons that are still surrounding both Hill and Winston in 2021. The team should once again have an RB1 in Kamara and a WR1 in Thomas.

NFC WEST

Lauren Carpenter

Seattle Seahawks Fantasy Preview

KEY LOSSES: Greg Olsen (TE)

KEY ADDITIONS: Gerald Everett (TE)

OFFSEASON FANTASY IMPACT: The Seahawks had a relatively quiet offseason on offense, but they did secure WR Tyler Lockett to a four-year contract extension. Gerald Everett is an intriguing addition for fantasy, given his production in Los Angeles with 41 receptions on 62 targets for 417 yards but only one touchdown.

NFL DRAFT PICKS OF FANTASY IMPACT: D'Wayne Eskridge (WR). The last thing that the Seahawks need is more weapons at wide receiver, but they used their first pick in the draft to add one. By trading away their 1st Round pick for Jamal Adams last year, the Seahawks did not select a player until the 56th overall pick. Eskridge can bring another deep threat option for QB Russell Wilson to target, which may eventually take away from Lockett and D.K. Metcalf.

OFFENSIVE OUTLOOK: The Seattle Seahawks were on fire last year until the wheels started falling off. Their defense was laughable, and Wilson struggled to remain upright. Still, it will be challenging to keep Wilson, Lockett, and Metcalf bottled up, and adding Everett in the offseason and Eskridge at the draft gives Wilson even more firepower to work with. A Metcalf-Wilson or Lockett-Wilson stack would give a fantasy team the upside to win weeks.

RB Chris Carson is returning for the 2021 season after playing 12 regular-season games and finishing with just over 680 yards on 141 attempts and only five touchdowns. Still, having Carson as an RB2 would be a solid addition to a fantasy roster with his consistency if he can stay on the field.

DEFENSIVE OUTLOOK: I won't mince words. Their passing defense needs some work. In 2020, they allowed the most completions in the NFL (450), on the most attempts (674), and the most plays (1,112). Defense against the run was better as they surrendered the fifth-fewest rushing yards (1,529) and the ninth-fewest rushing touchdowns (18). The Seahawks would be a solid contender to stream but are matchup dependent.

2021 TEAM OUTLOOK: Unless Seattle addresses their Swiss-Cheese offensive line, we will likely be looking at a near photocopy of last season. However, they have numerous high-upside fantasy pieces across the skill positions. Trade rumors were surrounding Wilson over the summer, but he remains a Seahawk, and Seattle is in a better place because of it.

Los Angeles Rams Fantasy Preview

KEY LOSSES: Jared Goff (QB), Malcolm Brown (RB), Josh Reynold (WR), Gerald Everett (TE)

KEY ADDITIONS: Matthew Stafford (QB)

OFFSEASON FANTASY IMPACT: Upgrading from Jared Goff to Matthew Stafford is a major fantasy progression. This QB change is a boost for every position in Los Angeles. Stafford is gritty and tough, having survived Detroit for 12 years. Despite a lack of pass-catchers last year, Stafford had 339 completions on 528 attempts for 4,084 yards and 26 touchdowns. Before he was injured in 2019, he was on pace for over 5,000 yards and 40 touchdowns.

NFL DRAFT PICKS OF FANTASY IMPACT: Tutu Atwell (WR). Atwell will be playing behind the one-two combo of Robert Woods and Cooper Kupp this season, but that doesn't mean he won't make an impact. His relevance for fantasy will likely be confined to deeper leagues, but the Rams no longer have Josh Reynolds or Gerald Everett competing with him for targets.

OFFENSIVE OUTLOOK: Having Stafford at the helm in Los Angeles is about as exciting as it can get for football fans who are eager to prove they are worthy of a Lombardi trophy after getting to the big dance and losing. Stafford's presence boosts all of the receivers, the running backs, and he can also be a solid option for fantasy on his own. Add that to the Woods-Kupp combo with a sprinkle of Tyler Higbee and a healthy dose of phenom Cam Akers, and there are fantasy options galore. If there is a piece available to take on the Rams, grab it. Everett vacates 62 targets in the passing game, and Reynolds adds another 81 possible (and conservative) number of targets up for grabs between Woods, Kupp, Atwell, and Higbee. They will benefit the most from Everett's absence.

Akers is primarily the line-from-scrimmage back, seeing only 14 targets over 13 games. He had a slow start to the season in his rookie year dealing with a committee backfield and an injury and didn't get rolling until Week 12. However, he exploded through Week 14 to emerge as the back to roster. Brown vacates 101 rush attempts that he turned into 419 yards and five touchdowns. However, Darrell Henderson is still around and rushed 138 times for 624 yards and five touchdowns last season over 15 games. Henderson will still play a part in the Rams offense, but Akers is the more exciting and productive player and the one to target in drafts.

DEFENSIVE OUTLOOK: If you didn't know, the Rams DST is consistently good. They ranked second in sacks with 53, and Aaron Donald was responsible for 13.5 of them. He was second behind T.J. Watt of the Pittsburgh Steelers with 15. Their pass defense, which includes Jalen Ramsey and Darious Williams, was also second in passing yards allowed with 1,406 behind the Washington Football Team. They are among the defense elites, totaling 123 points over the season and averaging a third-best 7.7 points a game.

2021 TEAM OUTLOOK: Much like the sun that shines down on the palm trees and beaches in LA, the future of the Rams is very, very bright. Stafford gives the entire team an immediate boost for 2021, and the Rams will provide fantasy points on both sides of the football and at every position.

Arizona Cardinals Fantasy Preview

KEY LOSSES: Kenyan Drake (RB), Dan Arnold (TE)

KEY ADDITIONS: James Conner (RB), A.J. Green (WR)

OFFSEASON FANTASY IMPACT: There isn't too much going on here with fantasy impact except for the situation at running back. Swapping out Kenyan Drake and grabbing James Conner isn't an upgrade, especially given the longevity concerns for James Conner. WR A.J. Green is a fun addition to the squad, but he is approaching his tenth year in the league and has lost much of his former "elite" status. Instead of hurting DeAndre Hopkins, Green's addition should help draw defenses and give the WR1 an even better chance at fantasy dominance in 2021.

NFL DRAFT PICKS OF FANTASY IMPACT: Rondale Moore (WR) has a fascinating home with the Arizona Cardinals as a slot receiver. Adding more weapons for QB Kyler Murray certainly doesn't hurt, but they now have a trustworthy slot guy in Moore who could make a name for himself in his rookie year.

OFFENSIVE OUTLOOK: There are so many great fantasy assets on the Cardinals, it's hard to know where to stop. The only position they are missing is a tight end, and neither Maxx Williams nor Darrell Daniels is the answer for fantasy purposes. However, having a piece of the Cardinals' offense could provide monster upside for your roster. Murray finished as the QB1 in 2020, just ahead of Josh Allen over 16 weeks, Hopkins finished as the WR4 in PPR, and even Kenyan Drake finished within the top-14.

The biggest question about Arizona's offense for fantasy is their running backs. Conner may be assuming the RB1 role and absorb a majority of Drake's 239 rush attempts. However, don't forget about Chase Edmonds. While he only saw 97 rush attempts with Drake last season, he was targeted 67 times for over 400 yards and four touchdowns. That was a drastic increase from his two prior seasons. Out of the two backs, I would aim for

Edmonds, who will have the better value in drafts and be used in the offense whether Conner is on the field or not.

DEFENSIVE OUTLOOK: Arizona's DST went on a run at the beginning of the year finishing within the top-10 five times out of the first seven weeks. They took a nose-dive after that but managed to pull out a few excellent performances at the end of the season. They had a few stinker weeks in juicy matchups, but overall are a good streaming option depending on the matchup. They finished 2020, tied for fourth with the Buccaneers with 48 sacks, and were third in tackles with 778.

2021 TEAM OUTLOOK: There is very little stopping the Cardinals from making an epic run in 2021. Murray has another year of experience and is hopefully healthy after the offseason while having excellent weapons surrounding him in the passing game. They are weakest at running back, but Murray himself is a dual-threat quarterback who can use his legs to the team's best advantage. If the defense can be more consistent, it can take some pressure off the offense.

San Francisco 49ers Fantasy Preview

KEY LOSSES: Jordan Reed (TE), Marquise Goodwin (WR)

KEY ADDITIONS: Trey Lance (QB - Rookie), Trey Sermon (RB - Rookie), Wayne Gallman (RB), Mohamed Sanu (WR)

OFFSEASON FANTASY IMPACT: TE Jordan Reed retired, but that isn't too impactful for fantasy since George Kittle is the dominant pass-catching force in San Francisco. True to HC Kyle Shanahan's modus operandi, there are even more mouths to feed among running backs. They added Wayne Gallman, signed Kyle Juszczyk to a five-year deal, and signed Jeff Wilson to a one-year contract extension. Mohamed Sanu is an exciting addition to the wide receiving corps and maybe an annoying target sniper instead of fantasy-relevant rosters.

NFL DRAFT PICKS OF FANTASY IMPACT: Trey Lance (QB), Trey Sermon (RB) While adding QB Trey Lance may not have an immediate impact for redraft in 2021, it does put a fire under Jimmy Garoppolo to compete for the starting job. Lance will likely stay on the bench for the 2021 season to learn behind Garoppolo if he can stay healthy.

Adding Trey Sermon to an already crowded backfield isn't great for his fantasy value, but that has become the norm for Shanahan. Unfortunately, Sermon will likely be swallowed up if he can't break out and make a name for himself early and stay healthy.

OFFENSIVE OUTLOOK: In addition to the draft day buzz, the 49ers will be heading into 2021 with a full roster of healthy players, which is a far cry from last year. If history is any judge, we may see Lance sooner rather than later if Garoppolo cannot remain upright. If Lance does indeed get the nod (whether by injury or not), it isn't ideal for their wide receivers such as Brandon Aiyuk, Deebo Samuel, James Richie, and newcomer Sanu. Of course, this isn't new, either. Aiyuk and Samuel will still be a threat in fantasy.

The running back situation doesn't get more "by committee" than in San Francisco. Legitimate starters include Raheem Mostert, Jeff Wilson, and Kyle Juszcyzk. After that, it could be a combination of those three-plus Gallman, Sermon, and maybe even JaMycal Hasty if Shanahan feels creative. Wilson may provide the best value in drafts out of all of the running backs, but his consistency (along with every other running back) is not guaranteed. So it will be difficult, yet again, to judge which back will be getting a full workload from week to week.

Then, of course, there's Kittle, who is unquestionably an elite tight end in the NFL and will finish in the top-3 at the end of the season. He battled injury last year but has an offseason to get healthy and dominate in the receiving game once again.

DEFENSIVE OUTLOOK: The 49ers DST ranked in the bottom half of fantasy finishers (depending on league scoring), but their lower rank isn't quite indicative of the week-to-week stream ability. They were either outstanding, or they were awful. They finished in the top-10 six times but also saw the bottom-10 six times. Nevertheless, they are strong contenders as a streaming option in the right matchup.

2021 TEAM OUTLOOK: The real buzz for the 49ers is Lance, who is the shiny new toy that likely won't be unboxed until 2022. The future is inspiring for San Francisco, but that may not come to fruition in 2021. Instead, the team will need to focus on staying healthy to unleash their true talent, power across the board.

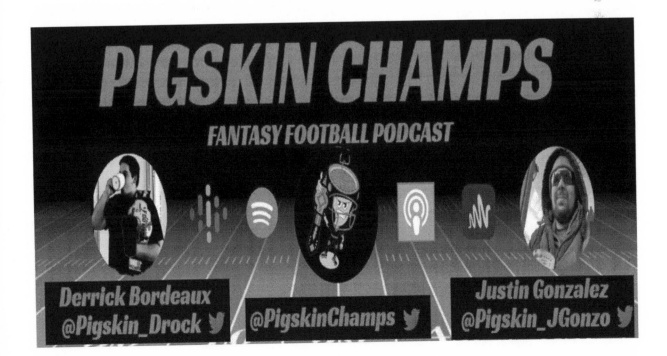

Chapter 13

NFL DFS 2021

Chris Meaney

DFS Intro

For me, DFS is all about finding value. I don't know what you do with your Sunday mornings, but I like to go bargain shopping for opportunity and volume. When I hosted *The FanDuel Show*, on FNTSY Sports Network, Joe Pisapia and I would create value lineups where we would only spend 75% of our budget. The goal wasn't to spend the least amount of money as possible, but to provide the viewers with a value play at each position, so they could afford studs in good spots.

I remember my first big call...a guest spot on the Fantasy Footballers podcast. It was the most ridiculous suggestion ever and after I finished my segment, I wondered if I really did suffer a concussion at hockey earlier that week. As you likely know by now, the tight end position in fantasy football is pitiful. You either spend up for Travis Kelce, George Kittle and Darren Waller or you look for value and spend down (punt) at the position.

I still remember Mike Wright asking if we should even bother with the tight end position because at that time, it was either you spent up for Rob Gronkowski or you took a shot with a much lesser name. I said "Well, the Oakland Raiders allowed 14 catches, 194 yards and four touchdowns to Crockett Gillmore and Tyler Eifert in their first two games. Gary Barnidge has six targets through two games, maybe there's something there." We all laughed. Awkwardly. I thought my fantasy football career was done. Barnidge entered career game number 72 that week and he only had 48 catches on his NFL resume. The Browns' tight end caught six of his 10 targets for 105 yards and he found the end zone that day. It led me to a co-hosting gig with the Fantasy Footballers DFS For the Rest of Us podcast.

Oddly enough, Barnidge went on to score four more touchdowns over his next three games. He crushed his previous career highs with 79 catches, 125 targets, 1,043 yards and nine touchdowns. It turns out it wasn't just about the Oakland Raiders - who allowed the most touchdowns to tight ends in 2015 - but it was about seeking out value through opportunity. Barnidge wasn't just called on for blocking that season as the Browns were limited with passing options and they played from behind often.

Later that year, I talked to Matt Forte - former Chicago Bears running back and big fantasy football player - about their game plan vs Oakland. I told him that in the daily fantasy community, word was out that the Raiders couldn't cover the TE and many were on Martellus Bennett having a big game. He chuckled and said "yeah, we knew...it's a copycat league." Bennett had a season-high 13 targets, 11 catches, 83 yards and a touchdown against Oakland.

Of course, the players are aware of what matchups they can exploit, but you need to be as well. It's very important to follow team trends, news, lines and totals throughout the year. You need to be on top of each team's tendencies. Which teams struggle to stop the run, which struggle against backs who catch, which get beat over the top or over the middle and which play at the fastest or slowest pace. Be on top of personnel change and you will be with the purchase of the Black Book.

Before we get into strategy and how to attack each position let's talk about the types of contests that are available to you. There are two separate types of games in daily fantasy sports: cash games and tournaments. I'll go over each game type and the differences between the two, including which strategies to take when building your lineups.

CASH GAMES

Cash game contests are the way to go if you're a new player in the DFS world. You don't need to ignore tournaments, but this is a great way to start and it doesn't require you to spend much. There are several people I know who started out playing multiple 25 cent contests each week. You don't need to score as much either as these contests are much smaller. The majority of cash games consist of contests such as head-to-heads, double-ups, triple-ups and 50/50s. In a head-to-head contest you only have to beat one other person. In a 50/50 contest, you must take down half of your competition to double your entry.

These contests are the easiest to earn a profit and maintain a bankroll throughout the season. That's if you play with little risk and roster the safest lineup as possible, because the playing field is much smaller in these types of contests. That's the goal here as you're not necessarily looking for upside. For example, a QB who likes to run and an RB who plays on a run heavy team provide a solid floor. They are considered safe cash game players as they provide little risk. Drafting a lineup of players who have a solid floor is the way to go. Tom Brady could get you two points on any given Sunday and he could also throw five touchdowns. If Lamar Jackson has a bad passing game, he could still return a profit with his rushing ability. There are more two-point games in Brady's outlook than Lamar's and even though he's not as good a passer as Brady, he's a safer QB in fantasy. Very rarely do I roster a QB who has zero rushing upside.

If you're a new player, don't go looking for head-to-head matchups, create them and let people join them. This way you are not joining one of the many possible leagues set up by experts. Also, look for beginner leagues as DraftKings has done a nice job over the past couple years catering to those who are just starting out.

GUARANTEED-PRIZE POOL TOURNAMENTS (GPP)

You can roster some of the same players in tournaments as you do in cash games, but you'll have to take somewhat of a different approach with the rest of your lineup if you want to have success. These contests are typically harder to win as you're competing against a larger group of people. The tougher the competition, the more satisfying it is when you win, though. Some of the prize pools in tournaments can be life changing.

When putting together your lineup, you still want to jump on value when possible, but overall, you're looking for upside plays. Imagine each player hitting their maximum potential, or at least close to it. In cash contests you're looking for a solid floor, but in tournaments you're looking for the highest ceiling. Your entire lineup doesn't need to be filled with only boom or bust players but think big when you're drafting. Unlike the cash contests, you'll need to finish near the top (17%-20%) to earn a profit.

It's important to try and take a different approach with your lineups in tournaments, by avoiding some of the obvious plays, which many in the industry call "chalk plays". If a player is in a good spot with a cheap price tag, it's certainly OK to roster that player, but know he'll probably have a high ownership number. You don't want to avoid all the high ownership players, but it's key to separate your roster from others in case that "for sure play" bombs. Projecting ownerships can go a long way and it sometimes means taking a contrarian approach with your roster. That could be as simple as taking a QB or WR in a bad matchup.

Be careful of which tournaments you enter. I typically don't like to go into tournaments where people can play hundreds of lineups. I like to enter a contest where the max is set at 3-5 per person. It eliminates a lot of randomness, which by the way is not a bad strategy if you play multiple lineups. Satellites are always worth your time if you're a big tournament spender as the reward can involve a trip along with a big payout or an entree to a bigger contest.

Quarterbacks

Quarterbacks typically rack up the most fantasy points, but that doesn't mean you need to spend up at the position every week. There's a ton of variation and the gap between QB1 and QB10 sometimes isn't that big at all. If you can get your QB to score three times the amount of his price tag you're off to a good start. If Jalen Hurts is $6,7K he would have to score 20.1 points to return a profit you want.

I typically shy away from the high-priced quarterbacks as I reserve my money for wideouts and backs. It doesn't mean I won't break the bank as it all depends on the matchups that week. Don't ignore an expensive quarterback if they are playing in a high total game, but make sure that game is going to be competitive. There's some risk in rostering a QB on a team who may win by 20 plus points. Sometimes targeting players on bad teams is a strategy to take. The Atlanta Falcons struggled on defense yet again in 2020 which resulted in a league-high 626 passing attempts from Matt Ryan. He has zero rushing upside, but he's loaded with weapons, he plays in a dome, and his defense will be one of the worst units again this season. His ceiling is tremendous.

Stacking a wide receiver and a quarterback is not a must but it's a strategy that works in cash and tournaments. You should mostly always want to match your QB with one of their favorite targets due to the correlation between the points their receivers will rack up. There's certainly a risk this strategy could flop, that's why it's one to take in tournaments. For the most part, if your WR has a good day, your QB will too. You want to maximize your full potential and stacking allows you to do that. There are certain quarterbacks like Jackson and Hurts who you could play solo because they could easily finish with zero passing touchdowns and two rushing scores. You hear the team "naked" in DFS and this is exactly what that means (Jackson and none of his weapons).

Stacking a running back with a quarterback is a contrarian approach you can take in tournaments. Stacking increases your variance and, although it's not the best strategy to take, I've seen millions get won from rosters only represented by one team. The first millionaire maker winner I saw had a team full of Pittsburgh Steelers.

Running Backs

A couple of things I like to look at when selecting my running backs are touches, carries, snaps, red zone usage and team implied totals. If the Los Angeles Rams are favored by 17.5 at home, I'll more likely lean towards Cam Akers than Matthew Stafford and Cooper Kupp. My feeling here is that the Rams will be up big, and they'll lean on Akers to run out the clock. Following spreads and game totals is a huge part of the DFS game.

If you're a FanDuel player, a back who isn't involved in the passing game isn't that big of a downgrade as it is on DraftKings where you get a full point for a catch. It's much harder to roster a running back who won't see the field if his team gets down in the game. Garbage time is real and three or four catches on a final drive goes a long way. Red zone rushing attempts are always an important stat to follow, but even more so if you're playing on FanDuel as you can take a risk on a back who doesn't catch a lot of balls because you only get half a point per reception.

Wide Receivers & Tight Ends

Targets are the name of the game when it comes to selecting wide receivers. Target shares, red zone targets, air-yards and the average depth of targets (aDOT) are things you should focus on heavily. You want to select wideouts who not only play for teams who like to throw the ball but like to throw it in the red zone. All of these statistics are tracked for free at FTN, including air-yards which has been a big part of my strategy over the past couple of seasons. I like to identify which players are receiving the most shots down the field and which QB's are taking those shots.

Wideouts who receive short targets benefit more on DraftKings where you get the full point for a catch. The deeper the target is, the greater the scoring ceiling. In tournaments, you should focus on wide receivers with a high scoring potential.

As mentioned above, the strategy for picking a tight end is simple, although it can be frustrating. There's nothing worse than spending up and getting a dud performance. Focus on tight ends who are part of the game plan, especially when their team gets inside the red zone.

DST

It's not always about attacking low scoring total games as I typically like to roster a DST who has the ability to create turnovers. Of course, the fewer points your DST allows the more fantasy points you'll get, but it's the turnovers that will set you apart.

That means attacking a team who will likely have their way on offense which will force the opposing team to step back and throw more than they may have liked heading into the game. A strong offense will allow the defense to dial up pressure which will relate to turnovers. Keeping in mind, you get a point for a sack and two points for fumbles recovered as well as interceptions. I typically like to spend down at defense, but if I have the money to spend up I will.

Scoring

DraftKings uses PPR scoring and rewards a three-point bonus for 100 yards rushing, 100 yards receiving and 300 yards passing, while FanDuel uses half point scoring.

Strategy & Tips

As you know, I like to find value and the best way to do that is to project targets and touches. Sometimes it's because an injury occurs, a matchup is sweet or a promotion up the depth chart. It's not always about picking players on the best teams although you want to maximize your ceiling.

The first thing I do each Tuesday morning when the schedule flips - before even looking at the price of players - is look at the matchups. I'm looking for opening lines and team implied totals. Vegas should have a huge influence on your thinking and construction of lineups. They don't build big buildings in Vegas for nothing. They have a pretty good idea of what's going on from week-to-week. It doesn't mean you have to agree with them but looking at totals and team implied totals will help you paint a picture of how you think each game will go.

Sometimes seeing the price of a player will influence how you feel about them, so I rank everyone before I look at price tags. Predicting a script is half the battle. If Bills and Ravens total is at 36.5, and you believe it'll be a low scoring game like Vegas has predicted, then there really isn't much of a point in rostering many from this contest. Maybe the backs or the DST's from this game and that's all.

Maybe the biggest tip of all is patience. Although you are spending money, don't let a bad week shake you up. There's so much variance in fantasy sports and losing streaks happen. You just have to accept them and be willing to move on. Recency bias is a thing so don't get caught up in it.

As mentioned earlier, don't get trapped into spending all of your money. It's OK to leave a few hundred off the board. Be aware of ownership projections (available at FTN), but don't ignore someone you like because you think they'll be chalky. The fantasy community is more in touch than ever and they can easily pump up a player who moves up a depth chart. Don't ignore public perception, but as my ol' buddy Joe says..."If it's right, it's right." This is just me, but I tend to stay away from average players who are talked up throughout the week.

There are a couple different ways you can look at ownerships. You can either side with the chalk or against it. Don't be afraid to be contrarian. You don't have to do this all the time, but if you like a QB atop the board, but you're afraid of spending all that money...it's likely others are too. On the flip side, don't be afraid to fade some of the talent atop the board. Look at games which will be played in a dome, have a unique lineup in tournaments, but most of all have fun! If you have any questions along the way, you can always reach me on Twitter @chrismeaney.

Chapter 14

NFL Wagering

Mike Randle

The NFL and Sports Betting is a perfect marriage. A weekly schedule combined with the unpredictability of a physical competition creates the precise balance of variables that entice millions of sports fans to search for ideal wagering opportunities.

There are multiple betting angles to explore with different strategies to help identify and maximize monetary value.

Here are my general wagering guidelines and four specific team total bets and three player bets I am looking to make before the upcoming 2021 NFL season.

I. NFL GAMBLING OVERVIEW:

Here are five tips to keep in mind as you prepare your wagers for the 2021 NFL Season.

Rule No. 1: Be Objective

In order to make sound betting decisions with positive EV (Expected Value) you need to remain completely objective as a bettor. We all have predetermined allegiances to a favorite team or player, but each game is its own independent entity and should be examined as such. Before the season begins, become self-aware of your ingrained biases and analyze your ability to stay neutral. If you have a strong allegiance to a certain team, it may be best to avoid betting them completely.

Rule No. 2: Remember The Importance of Home Field Advantage

It is wonderful that fans will be able to return to the games for the 2021 season. Playing in front of empty stadiums last year decreased home field advantages across the league. Last season, teams posted a losing record at home for the first time since the NFL-AFL merger. Here are NFL home win rates for the past three seasons, per USA Today:

- 2018: 60.6%
- 2019: 51.8%
- 2020: 49.8%

There was also a significant difference in the betting market. Using data from BetLabs, home favorites only covered at a 45.9% rate (67-79), as opposed to a 48.4% (1407-1502-89) success rate since 2003.

We would expect home field advantage to return in 2021, making last year's best home cover teams even stronger.

- Miami Dolphins (7-1)
- Buffalo Bills (6-2)
- Seattle Seahawks (6-2)

Being aware of the return of home field advantage could be a profitable investment early in the season, if the books haven't adjusted properly to the anomaly of last season.

Rule No. 3: Late Season Divisional Games? Bet The Under

Familiarity breeds contempt.

NFL teams are always focused on achieving dominance within their own division. When a team plays a divisional opponent late in the season, it often is a close game. Over the past seven seasons, December divisional underdogs have covered the spread at a 54.6% rate (118-98-6), with a 6.6% ROI. If you remove the only season (2017-2018) where the home favorite actually had a winning record, the underdog cover rate jumps to 57.6% (102-75-6). Regardless of season performance, divisional games late in the season are usually close, which provides the savvy bettors with prime wagering opportunities.

Rule No. 4: Monitor Injury Reports

Injuries play a crucial role in handicapping an NFL game. For example, an injury to a key offensive linemen for a road underdog can play a critical role in the efficiency of that team's offense. Always take note of star players who leave a game because of injury, and evaluate whether the opening line for the following week reflects that player possibly missing the subsequent game. This is particularly true for teams with a short turnaround to a Thursday night game.

Rule No. 5: Situational Spots

There are times during the season where underdogs tend to give their best effort. One of those times is as a winless home team during Week 3. Over the past three seasons, teams that are 0-2 as a home underdog in Week 3 are 6-2 (75%) against the spread with a ROI of 42.1%. Only six teams since 1980 have made the playoffs after starting 0-3, making for live home underdogs after two consecutive losses to start the season.

II. NFL Over/Under Win Totals

There are a myriad of available wagers from several different websites and casinos. Here is a closer look at my favorite Team Total Bets for the upcoming season.

Denver Broncos Over 8.5 Wins: I think Denver hits this over regardless of who is at quarterback. Prior to this year's NFL Draft, the Broncos ranked as the sixth-best roster per PFF. Head coach Vic Fangio is a defensive wizard, and will benefit from the healthy return of pass rushers Bradley Chubb and Von Miller. Needing to compete with the explosive passing games of the Chiefs and Chargers, the Broncos also prioritized bolstering an already strong pass defense. Denver signed Kyle Fuller and Ronald Darby in the offseason and drafted Alabama cornerback Patrick Surtain to fortify the best secondary in the NFL.

The Broncos have surrounded quarterback Drew Lock with explosive receiving weapons. Courtland Sutton returns after missing most of the 2020 season (torn ACL), and looks to regain his 2019 form when he tallied 72 receptions, 1112 receiving yards, and six receiving touchdowns. Fellow wide receivers Tim Patrick (51 receptions), Jerry Jeudy (113 targets), and KJ Hamler (4.32 speed), all flashed big-play ability last season.

Denver's best receiver is one of the NFL's best tight ends, Noah Fant, who ranked third at the position with 383 yards after catch.

The Broncos moved up in the draft to select versatile running back Javonte Williams, who comps to former Denver standout RB Knowshon Moreno (PlayerProfiler). He provides depth to two-time Pro Bowler rusher Melvin Gordon, behind a healthy and improved Denver offensive line.

Denver has a schedule advantage with nine home games in the altitude at Mile High Stadium, including very winnable games against the Jets and Lions. Add in a road game against Jacksonville, and Denver should have three predictable wins excluding divisional play.

If the Aaron Rodgers trade rumors materialize, this line should go to nine or even 9.5 games. I believe in the Broncos talent and superior coaching, and love the upside if somehow Rodgers joins the team in August or even September.

Minnesota Vikings Over 8.5 Wins: The Packers were the overwhelming favorite to win their third consecutive NFC North title, but have seen their odds drop over the past month as the Rodgers drama has increased.

Under the guidance of defensive-minded head coach Mike Zimmer, the Vikings ranked third and fourth in defensive DVOA in the 2018 and 2019 seasons. As a result of injuries and poor performance, the Vikings finished just 18th in DVOA last season, including an embarrassing 30th in run defense per FootballOutsiders. Zimmer will now have a refreshed and replenished defense that should again ascend to the top of the league.

Defensive lineman Danielle Hunter returns from a neck injury, and hopes to regain his 18-sack form from the 2019 season. Michael Pierce opted out last season and combined with the signing of Dalvin Tomlinson (6-foot-3, 318 lbs), Minnesota should have one of the NFC's best defensive fronts.

The Vikings secondary added eight-time Pro Bowler Patrick Peterson to start opposite All-Rookie Team CB Cameron Dantzler.

Minnesota's eighth-most efficient offense features playmakers at every skill position. Wide receivers Justin Jefferson and Adam Thielen balance a strong rushing attack behind RB Dalvin Cook. Minnesota also made improving the offensive line a top priority with the addition of first-round tackle Christian Darrisaw of Virginia Tech, and Ohio State guard Wyatt Davis in Round 3.

If the Packers trade Aaron Rodgers, Minnesota becomes the favorite in the NFC North. The Vikings should greatly improve on their 7-9 record from last season, and Zimmer's improved defense makes them a great division bet in the NFC North

Houston Texans Under 4.5 Wins: I hope this total is still available at the time of publication. The Deshaun Watson uncertainty is the nail in the coffin on what should be a terrible season for the Texans. Assuming a sweep of Jacksonville (not guaranteed), it is difficult to find three more wins on the Houston schedule. The Texans' out of division games include the NFC West, AFC East, a road game at Cleveland, and two home games against the Chargers and Panthers.

There is massive turnover across the roster including the coaching staff. First-time head coach David Culley is tasked with structuring a defense that brought in 16 new players *prior* to the NFL Draft. On offense, the Texans are filled with aging veterans lacking explosiveness such as 29-year old RB David Johnson and 30-year old wide receiver Randall Cobb. If Watson does, in fact, miss games, the Texans get even older with 31-year old Tyrod Taylor under center.

Coming off a 4-12 season, without future Hall of Famer J.J. Watt, having a new head coach, aging offense, new personnel on defense, and having no first or second round draft pick, the Texans are one of my favorite under bets in the 2021 season. I would even consider taking this down to 4 or potentially 3.5 wins.

Philadelphia Eagles Under 6.5 Wins: Philadelphia parted ways with former head coach Doug Pederson and hired former Indianapolis offensive coordinator Nick Sirianni as his replacement. The Eagles have also made a full change at quarterback from Carson Wentz to 22-year old Jalen Hurts. There is certainly long-term potential for Philadelphia, but in a very competitive NFC East division I think they go under this total in 2021.

Philadelphia finished last season ranked 15th in defensive DVOA per FootballOutsiders, including a disappointing 24th against the pass. The Eagles completely overhauled the defense, losing DT Malik Jackson, DE Vinny Curry, LB Nate Gerry, CB Nickell Robey-Coleman, and safety Jalen Mills.

The Eagles brought in an influx of new offensive personnel from the draft and free agency, but will likely experience growing pains with Hurts as quarterback. The impact of explosive players such as rookie wideout DeVonta Smith will be tethered to the overall success of the offense. With the Giants and Washington both possessing strong defensive fronts, and Dallas having one of the league's best offensive attacks, it will be an uphill battle for the Eagles.

The last challenge Philadelphia faces is with their schedule. In the first six weeks, the Eagles will travel to Atlanta and Dallas, and host San Francisco, Kansas City, and the defending Super Bowl champion Buccaneers.

As a result of inexperience at head coach, quarterback, a poor defense, and challenging schedule, I'm taking the Eagles Under 6.5 wins.

III. Off-Season Specials

Taysom Hill Week 1 New Orleans Starting Quarterback +145: What, exactly, is the logic that Jameis Winston is starting for the Saints in Week 1? When the Saints were 7-2 with Super Bowl aspirations, head coach Sean Payton chose Taysom Hill over Winston last season. New Orleans went 3-1 in Hill's starts.

In a league that places a huge premium on rushing quarterbacks, Hill is a better option to guide a Saints offense post-Drew Brees. On a New Orleans team with a superior defense and limited receiving weapons, it seems unlikely that the interception-prone Winston (30 interceptions in 2019) would be the best choice to guide the Saints towards an NFC Championship. The juice on this line is favorable due to the rumors of beat reporters, but as we saw with the Mac Jones/Trey Lance drama, don't be afraid to be contrarian to media reports and take advantage of favorable betting lines.

Najee Harris Offensive Rookie of the Year +800: While NFL MVP award tends to go to a quarterback, the Offensive Rookie of the Year has actually been the opposite in recent years. In the eight years since 2013, the award has gone to a non-QB player five times. At 6-foot-1, 232 lbs, the versatile Harris has the tools to be Pittsburgh's three-down bell cow. Steelers' head coach Mike Tomlin has a preference for one lead running back, and the first-round draft capital ensures Harris will get a strong look as the opening week starter. With a 90th percentile college target share at Alabama per PlayerProfiler, Harris is a better all-around option than Benny Snell or Anthony McFarland. This is a very enticing bet at 8 to 1 odds.

Russell Wilson NFL MVP +1600: Did we all forget that Wilson was the dominant leader for this award at the halfway point of last season? While the remainder of the season was a disappointment, Wilson's talent is not debatable. He still has two superior wideouts in DK Metcalf and Tyler Lockett, who combined for 183 receptions last season. Wilson entered last season at 8 to 1, and has now seen those odds double in 2021. I'm still a believer in Wilson, especially at this betting value.